CW01401988

e-Patients Live Longer

e-Patients Live Longer

The Complete Guide to Managing Health Care Using Technology

NANCY B. FINN

iUniverse, Inc.
Bloomington IN

e-Patients Live Longer
The Complete Guide to Managing Health Care Using Technology

iUniverse books may be ordered through booksellers or by contacting:

iUniverse
1663 Liberty Drive
Bloomington, IN 47403
www.iuniverse.com
1-800-Authors (1-800-288-4677)

ISBN: 978-1-4620-3038-5 (sc)
ISBN: 978-1-4620-3039-2 (hc)
ISBN: 978-1-4620-3040-8 (ebk)

Library of Congress Control Number: 2011910363

Printed in the United States of America

iUniverse rev. date: 09/10/2011

This book is about empowering every patient through technology and applications, which are the basis for health-care delivery in future generations.

It is dedicated to my grandchildren: Gefen, Alex, Marc, and Sydney Finn, who are empowered in so many ways and who are the future.

Foreword

" . . . communication extends all the way from the intimate interaction between a clinician and a patient, to the most public dissemination of information."

Harvey Fineberg, MD, PhD
President, Institute of Medicine

Communication has been and always will be at the heart of healthcare. For most of the profession's history, physicians could do very little useful for patients but listen to them and offer them advice. Yet physicians who communicated effectively and compassionately well were still generally revered.

These same communication skills are arguably more important today, despite (or perhaps because of) the proliferation of technologies physicians can effectively apply to alleviate pain and suffering and prolong life. And yet, physicians often forget about these skills, due to the pressures of seeing ever more patients in decreasing amounts of time. Because of these pressures, physicians have increasingly focused on regurgitating facts and ordering tests, rather than spending time talking and listening to their patients.

But communication with patients is critical to patient engagement. Patient engagement in the care process results in greater satisfaction, better adherence to care plans, improved outcomes, and consequently reduced healthcare costs. Although these costs savings do not accrue to the physicians in a fee-for-service world, they could ultimately result in improved reimbursements (especially true as we move to newer payment models). So ironically, the same financial pressures that are preventing physicians from taking the time to listen to their patients could be alleviated through better communication with their patients. In other words, investing time in connecting with patients pays dividends.

But the quality of communication is but one aspect. The tools we use to communicate are also important. Historically, all communication between patients and physicians took place in-person. But with the advent of the telephone in the early 20th century, physicians and patients learned how to best apply this technology, for the betterment of patient care. Today there are many other ways we can connect with patients, including electronic messaging of various types, video conferencing, using telemedicine, and now social networking. But physicians have been reluctant to adopt these technologies, despite their apparent benefits, for a variety of reasons (some legitimate and many not). Even relatively low-tech tools like e-mail, which burst on the popular scene with the advent of the World Wide Web in the mid-1990s, is still shunned by the majority of physicians, despite guidelines that were published over a decade ago. If we are to create a scalable healthcare system to manage the increasing care needs of our expanding and aging population, we must expand our notions of patient-physician care beyond visit-based care; we must adopt additional communication technologies and optimize the selection based on the clinical situation being discussed, the availability of technologies, and the preference of those communicating.

The third element that relates to communication is a shift in mindset, both on the part of the patient and the physician, to make healthcare more effective. Patients must take responsibility for their health, and must recognize that healthcare is not a spectator sport, it is a participatory sport. They should participate in decision making with their physicians, ask questions, and be willing to invest time and effort in understanding their conditions. Physicians, for their part, must be willing to share information with their patients (including access to their records), and must respect that although they may be experts in some aspect of healthcare, their patients will always be experts in themselves. Moreover, they must encourage their patients to learn more about their disease and engage them in the development of shared care plans. They should not fear but should encourage patients as they evolve into e-patients: those that are **e**quipped, **e**nabled, **e**mpowered, and **e**ngaged.

In this book, Nancy Finn—a writer, editor, and consultant with a strong background in digital communication technology—explains why it is important to be an e-patient, and discusses the tools that facilitate patient engagement. She brings relevance to provider tools such as e-prescribing, electronic medical records, and health information exchanges, and even reviews advanced technologies that are in early stages of adoptions, such as telemedicine and home monitoring. Along the way, she discusses our sometimes dysfunctional healthcare system and how e-patients can leverage these technologies to overcome deficiencies in the system and improve their healthcare.

Technology is important and interesting, but is not an end unto itself. It is an enabler of new models of care and can lower barriers to patient engagement. That is why this book is so important to modern healthcare consumers. It is my sincere hope that through books like this that every patient will be an e-patient.

Daniel Z. Sands, MD, MPH

Senior Medical Informatics Director,

Cisco Internet Business Solutions Group

Assistant Clinical Professor of Medicine,

Harvard Medical School

Staff Physician,

Beth Israel Deaconess Medical Center

President,

Society for Participatory Medicine

Introduction

Profile of an e-Patient

Most people would agree that health care is a top priority. However, given the routines of daily life, planning and preparing for health issues are secondary to other pressures until there is a serious health concern to address. *E-Patients Live Longer* provides sound advice on how you can become an educated and empowered health consumer before being confronted by a major health crisis. This book explains what it is like to be an e-Patient who uses the electronic communication technology that you use every day, including e-mail, the Internet, and wireless mobile devices such as smartphones and, tablets to communicate with your health-care team and have the information you need readily available. The book helps you understand digital health records and other information tools to insure that your personal health information is always right there, no matter where or when you might need care. The book wades through the maze of online resources, suggests the best routes for finding answers to your health-care questions, and helps you to engage with other patients in online communities and social networking sites.

E-Patients Live Longer also describes how, using telemedicine technology, patients who live in remote areas can obtain second opinions, get expert trauma services, and receive consults from renowned specialists at major medical centers while remaining in your home. Those of you who suffer from chronic conditions will learn about technologies that enable you or a member of your family to monitor your condition via the Internet twenty-four-seven using computers, telephone lines, cameras, robotics, and other digital devices. You will also learn how medications can be ordered electronically and how your medication lists and medical history can be stored in a personal online file, eliminating so many of the mistakes that cause adverse reactions, medical errors, and death.

Most significantly, *e-Patients Live Longer* provides guidelines and suggestions for becoming an empowered patient who comes to the doctor's office with the right list of questions to get the answers you need; engaging your health-care providers in a dialogue via e-mail and e-visits; overseeing the privacy of your health information; and evaluating which health plan will most effectively meet your needs and those of your family.

The term "e-Patient" was coined by Dr. Tom Ferguson in 1975. "Dr. Tom," as he was known, was an author, physician, and researcher who led the movement for collaboration between patients and health-care professionals. In a 2007 white paper entitled *"E-Patients: How They Can Help Us Heal Healthcare,"* Dr. Tom wrote:

> Millions of knowledge workers are emerging as unexpected health-care heroes. When they or a loved one become ill, they turn into e-Patients—citizens with health concerns who use the Internet as a health resource, studying up on their own diseases (and those of friends and family members), finding better treatment centers and insisting on better care, providing other patients with invaluable medical assistance and support, and increasingly serving as important collaborators and advisors for their clinicians (Thomas Ferguson, MD, with the e-Patients Scholars Working Group, March 2007).

E-Patients Live Longer is filled with suggestions, resources, and thought-provoking anecdotal stories that explain why health information technology and participatory medicine is so important and how to use it to protect yourself and insure that you are receiving the best possible care. This book is based on hundreds of interviews with individuals who are on the cutting edge of e-health and medical practice. It outlines exciting developments such as robotics, personalized medicine, and new health delivery infrastructures—including medical homes, community health-care centers, outpatient retail clinics, e-visits, telemedicine, and home monitoring—that will shape the future of health care. These are new opportunities and discoveries that will prolong your life while reinforcing your quality of care. This book points out what e-Patients can expect to see and how they can take advantage of exciting developments in health care.

Nancy Finn is a technologist, teacher, and communicator whose lifelong work has been to study, teach, and write about how communication technology affects social behavior. In e-*Patients Live Longer*, she brings her expertise into the health-care arena, where she shows how collaboration and communication can resolve many of the health-care issues we face as we attempt to care for aging populations with fewer resources and limited funds. Finn advocates for bringing the empowered patient into the health-care decision process. She argues that patients and the medical establishment must invest in communication technology, and she provides down-to-earth, common-sense solutions that readers can adopt. Individuals who must read this book include:

Baby boomers: People born in the U.S. in the post-World War II period from 1946 through 1964 number approximately seventy-five million individuals. You straddle between the two extremes of caring for yourselves and your children, while at the same time caring for your elderly parents. At both ends of the spectrum, you are faced with an onslaught of health-care issues. This book provides answers for your role as a health-care consumer and health-care advocate for elderly parents, spouses, and children.

Senior citizens: Over thirty-six million Americans are categorized as senior citizens, individuals over the age of sixty-five. You experience new and frightening illnesses as you age. You are already using the Internet for researching many topics, including health information. You use e-mail, and many of you have smartphones. You will find this book's concrete suggestions about where to find reliable, credible health information on the Internet invaluable. You will benefit from the book's discussions about privacy, health-care costs, telemedicine, and especially home monitoring systems. You will read with interest the tips and suggestions throughout the book, particularly ideas on how to choose a doctor or a hospital and the guidelines for patient safety.

Individuals with chronic conditions: There are over 133 million Americans of all ages who suffer from chronic conditions. You will learn about the value of digital health records, patient portals, telemedicine, the medical home, and how you can use the Internet to help manage your conditions. You will also benefit from the discussions about how to improve communication with health-care providers and descriptions of the digital tools available to help you access medical services twenty-four-seven to monitor your conditions.

The Patient who wants to morph into an e-Patient: Finally, this book is for everyone who will meet a health issue somewhere along the journey through life. You need to understand how to become an empowered, participatory patient who uses technology for health care that you use every day to conduct business, communicate with friends, engage in social networks, and research important topics online.

Content Disclaimer: The anecdotal stories sprinkled throughout the book are composites of several real patient stories that were relayed to the author or are from other publications and used with permission as noted in the endnotes.

Medical Disclaimer: This book is not a book about your health, specific diseases, or how to find the right cures or treatments. It is a book about how to use digital communication tools to empower yourself as a patient for better, safer health care.

CONTENTS

Chapter One

Power Up and Communicate with Your Health-Care Providers

Be what you are and say what you feel because those who mind don't matter, and those who matter, don't mind.

Bennett Cerf, <u>Shake Well Before Using: A New Collection of Impressions and Anecdotes Mostly Humorous</u> (1948) p. 249.

The Patient Experience

Jim has asthma. At his office visit, he tells Dr. Oakes, his primary care physician (PCP) of fifteen years, that despite faithfully taking medications prescribed, he is wheezing a lot at night and sometimes awakens short of breath. Dr. Oakes reviews Jim's electrocardiogram (EKG), finds it to be normal, and listens carefully to Jim's heart and lungs. Everything seems to be fine. While Jim waits, Dr. Oakes searches Jim's records to locate his list of medications. They talk for a few minutes about what could be causing this problem. Dr. Oakes hands Jim a new prescription, which Jim will take to the pharmacy to fill. Dr. Oakes also writes orders for a chest X-ray and a pulmonary function test and suggests that Jim return in a month to review the results of these tests and his blood work. All of this paperwork takes time away from the all too short visit, which lasts a total of fifteen minutes.

This is a typical encounter between a physician and a patient. With time restrictions on doctors imposed by insufficient primary care reimbursement and a paper record system that takes the doctor several minutes to search, this office visit is structured so that there is barely time for Dr. Oakes to properly examine Jim. There is never enough time to formulate an evidence-based diagnosis and discuss a treatment plan, let alone talk to Jim about what else is on his mind. Dr. Oakes also writes his comments as they talk, so he is not able to give his full attention to what Jim is saying. The experience is frustrating for both Dr. Oakes and for Jim.

Sandra, a retired teacher with hypertension, has been a patient of Dr. Clarke for twenty years. When Sandra arrives for her annual visit, she is given a clipboard with a paper form that asks her to list all of her medications and fill in her medical history. She observes that this is the same form she filled out last year, as she diligently tries to remember all of the details required. Sandra is escorted into the exam room by a nurse who asks about her general health; checks Sandra's vitals; gets her weight; draws blood and does an EKG—all part of the routine annual checkup. When Dr. Clarke comes in, she greets Sandra, quickly glances at her update form, and reviews a piece of paper that Sandra has brought with her that has a list of blood pressure results Sandra has tracked over the past several weeks. They talk briefly about headaches that Sandra has been experiencing. After a quick but thorough examination, Dr. Clarke asks Sandra to get dressed and meet her in her office, where she sits at a computer terminal reviewing Sandra's electronic health record. With her eyes on the screen, Dr. Clarke tells Sandra that the exam was fine. She asks Sandra to continue tracking her blood pressure and send a weekly e-mail to the nurse, who will review the data for anything unusual. She enters a prescription for the headaches into the computer, which automatically checks the new medication for interactions with other medicines that Sandra is taking and sends the information electronically to Sandra's pharmacy. Dr. Clarke suggests that Sandra schedule another appointment in six months or sooner if the headaches persist or if there are any other problems. She encourages Sandra to e-mail her if she has further specific questions about the treatment plan.

This office visit, which also lasts approximately fifteen minutes, is a little closer to what a twenty-first century e-Patient visit with the doctor looks like. Sandra's information is in an electronic health record, and her doctor uses e-prescribing to send Sandra's medication to the pharmacy, reducing the possibility of medical errors from illegible handwritten prescriptions and insuring a more comprehensive check of drug interactions. The fact that Sandra is monitoring her blood pressure empowers Sandra to be more involved in her health care and, hopefully, this will keep her stable and out of the emergency room. Although the visit is pleasant and efficient, it does not foster the kind of communication and discussion that physicians and patients should routinely experience. The doctor is rushed. She is facing the computer and has her back to Sandra while they talk, so there is little eye contact and personal dialogue. The use of digital technology is a step in the right direction; however, the technology can be intrusive. Although Sandra has a way to connect with her physician between visits, which helps her adhere more rigorously to her physician's recommendations, there are things about their interaction that are unsettling.

What Do You Want From Your Visit with Your Doctor?

When you go to the doctor, you are seeking solutions to specific health issues. You want to be able to talk with your doctor, to feel welcomed, and to be assured that your issues are going to be addressed with respect, competence, and confidentiality. Here are suggestions regarding what to look for:

- A doctor who gives you his or her full attention and listens to what you have to say.
- A doctor who is thorough in examining you and checking your medications, blood pressure, heart, lungs, etc.
- Someone who is caring and compassionate and with whom you have a rapport that enables you to talk freely about your concerns.
- A doctor who is committed to helping you solve your health issues in the most efficient and effective way possible by offering communication channels beyond the limitations of the office visit.
- A physician who outlines all of your options for treatment and directs you to information resources on the Internet or articles that give you more detail than can be covered during the office visit.
- A physician who provides you with specific well-explained guidelines to follow when you leave the office.

What Makes You a Good Patient?

Doctors are human, health care is complex, and time spent with each patient is restricted. As an e-Patient, you must assume an appropriate level of responsibility for your care. You should come to the office visit prepared to provide a complete list of medications that you are currently taking, as well as up-to-date information on other providers you have seen and issues you have been dealing with. You must ask for explanations and guidance when your doctor's diagnosis or orders are confusing or contradictory. You must follow through with those orders, including taking and finishing all medications in the manner they are prescribed and complying with your doctor's request to keep records of your blood pressure or blood sugar. It is important to be forthright, even if it involves embarrassing personal issues. You should come to your annual checkup equipped with a pen and paper to write down comments that are difficult to remember during the visit. Some of the questions you might want to ask and answers you should record include:

- What do you think is causing my symptoms?
- What does this mean?
- Do I need tests?
- What kind of tests?
- When and how will I receive the test results?
- What are my treatment options?
- Do I want to see a specialist and why?
- Do I need medication?
- What kind of medication?
- What are the side effects of the medication?
- Are there lifestyles changes that I need to consider?
- When should I see you again? Can I ask you questions via e-mail?
- Can I view my test results?

Effective doctor-patient communication is critical to the delivery of appropriate health care. Your relationship with your medical provider and your interactions during the clinical encounter can influence your medical outcome and your satisfaction with your care. Open dialogue is based upon your doctor taking the time to listen to you, and your providing honest and complete information. There is no holding back information on drugs that you are taking, both prescription and over the counter. Your physicians need full, factual information about you in order to make a proper diagnosis. With both Jim and Sandra, the rushed encounter left little time for either patient to chat about their current life situation, their stress, their feelings, or other concerns that could have a serious impact on their health.

Studies of asthma patients reveal that when it comes to taking the oral steroids that are often essential for controlling asthma, many patients do not follow the doctor's directions for taking the medication. This is often due to the fact that these patients did not have the opportunity to discuss fully with their physician the reasons why they need medication, what is an appropriate dosage, and when and how to take the medication. (Inhalers can be very different from one another in the way they deliver a dose of medicine). As a result, the patients ignore the doctor's orders. Although they typically fill the prescription, they take their dosage erratically and often stop the medication completely after a few weeks or months. Eventually they end up back at the doctor's office or in the emergency room. Simple communication could help resolve this problem of noncompliance and keep patients more stable and able to control the disease. (1)

According to the Centers for Disease Control and Prevention (CDC), doctor visits in the United States have increased twenty percent in the last five years to more than 1.2 billion visits annually, while the number of primary care doctors across the country is falling. Each of these visits requires an intricate patchwork of information processing and communication. Most medical records are still on paper, (only about one-quarter of physicians have electronic records), although the Federal Stimulus bill passed in 2009 mandated doctors to implement electronic health records by 2014. It will be years beyond that before there is full meaningful use of digital health records, because it is a difficult and costly transition for physicians. Among physicians who do store their records in computer systems, most cannot exchange patient data electronically with other providers that you might see, widening the information gap in your care. As a result, your paperwork sits in isolated files in the possession of a myriad of providers, including your primary care physician, your specialists, hospitals where you have been admitted, labs where your blood and other tests are sent, physical and occupational therapists, alternative medicine specialists, your pharmacy, your dentist, and your health insurer.

In a study conducted by the Agency for Healthcare Research and Quality (AHRQ), which is a part of the Department of Health and Human Services, clinicians reported that in a representative sample of over 1,500 clinical visits, important information was missing in 13.6 percent of the cases. Among these visits, the most common missing information was lab and radiology results (45 percent and 28.2 percent, respectively), letters or dictation containing clinical information (39.5 percent), and patient history or physical exam findings (26.8 percent). When your physician does not have all of the facts, serious consequences can occur, including the need for expensive repeat tests or the possibility of medical error. (2)

Time, Tools, Teamwork

Talking to your doctor requires time, tools, and teamwork. You typically spend more of your day communicating (using the telephone, written word, and computer, or talking with other people) than in any other single activity. These habits provide a unique set of well-developed communication and listening skills. When it comes to your health care, those skills matter. More than 80 percent of the information that your doctor needs to make a correct diagnosis comes from what you say and your medical history. The rest comes from the examination and test results. Unless you accurately describe your problem, it is difficult for the doctor to determine what is wrong. Greater use of digital communication tools—electronic health records, e-mail, electronic databases, patient portals and e-visits (covered in more detail in chapters 2, 3, and 7)—could make a vital difference in assisting your physician in making a more accurate diagnosis and prescribing a treatment, enabling you and your physician to establish a better dialogue. Sending a medical history update form to your doctor in advance of your visit enables your physician to have all of the required information about you. Communicating with your providers more frequently between visits, for non-urgent issues, frees up time for you and your physician to address critical issues during the clinical visit.

Diana is a fifty-seven-year-old consultant who suffers from chronic arthritis and related autoimmune problems. Ten days before her scheduled visit, Diana receives an e-mail from her PCP's office with a link to the portal that Dr. Cooper shares with her patients. The e-mail reminds Diana to go to her private section of the portal and enter any recent problems, test results, or meetings with medical specialists or therapists she has had since her last visit. Early on the day of her appointment, an automated computer program sends a checklist of all the patients on her schedule to Dr. Cooper's smartphone. Just before Diana's visit, Dr. Cooper is able to quickly glance at Diana's portal entries and determine the agenda for their visit. When Diana arrives at the office, she goes directly to a computer terminal, where she scans her medical card. This notifies the staff that she has arrived and brings up her electronic health record. She is escorted to an examining room, where a nurse takes her vitals and keys that information directly into her the record. She leaves that screen visible for Dr. Cooper, who is able to look very quickly at the computer screen to assess Diana's condition. As a result, Dr. Cooper can focus on Diana without the distraction of having to look up information. Dr. Cooper changes a couple of Diana's medications and sends a prescription directly from her computer to the pharmacy. She also sends an e-mail to Diana's rheumatologist to update him and posts links to Diana's patient portal site with her next appointment, all in a matter of seconds. Dr Cooper reminds Diana that if she has any questions, she can send her an e-mail. On her way out, Diana goes to a kiosk where a short survey is on the screen that asks a few questions about her satisfaction with the visit.

The Empowered Patient

Becoming an e-Patient requires you to change your philosophy regarding your health care. Instead of viewing the doctor as the guardian of your care, you must become an integral a part of the medical team taking care of you. There are several actions that will empower you:

- Do not stay with the same doctor if he or she is not meeting your needs. Choose a doctor who uses best practices in diagnosing and treating your problems.
- Gather a health-care team with whom you can collaborate to address your health concerns. Be sure there is two-way discussion about your health-care options.

- Assume responsibility for collecting your health history, test results, and provider notes, and bring that data with you when you meet with your physicians.
- Always arrive at your health-care provider's office with a list of issues prioritized according to what is most important to you.
- Elevate the quality and efficiency of your interactions with your health-care providers at each visit and set clear expectations regarding what you expect.
- Insist on fast access to medical attention when you have a serious problem, including same-day visits, whether online or in person.
- Seek advice and information on appropriate Internet resources to help you understand your problems, issues, medication side effects, and treatment options.
- Understand your health insurance choices.
- Arrange for a patient advocate when you are too ill to be your own advocate.
- Speak up when you are uncomfortable with what your physician might or might not be doing.

Talking to your doctors and getting what you need requires you to participate fully and take personal actions. You also need to protect yourself from shoddy care, medical error and overpayment. Here are a few questions to ask:

- How experienced is my doctor?
- Does he or she satisfy my needs?
- Do I need to see a specialist?
- What hospital best fits my needs? Is it the big academic medical center forty miles away or the community hospital that is walking distance from my home?
- Is there a difference in what I would pay for a procedure or operation at these institutions?
- Does the difference align with the level of quality I might experience?
- Does my doctor provide me with options for treatment when appropriate?
- Does my doctor take the time to discuss my medications and help me understand all of the side effects and ways to take the medicine?
- Does my doctor help me find worthwhile web resources?

Key Points

1. In the fifteen-minute office visit, there is not enough time to discuss the complex issues that most patients bring with them. Alternative communications are necessary to provide your doctor with information in advance of the appointment. These communication systems also enable you to talk with your doctor or nurse after the appointment and to clear up unanswered questions and issues that arise. Options include planned Q&A online sessions with your doctor following the visit and e-mail queries sent to a qualified health-care professional who will answer your concerns.

2. Good communication includes honest, complete information that is free of jargon and involves good listening skills by both doctors and patients. Consider what might have changed in your life over the past several months to warrant communicating with your provider. Think of ways to improve communication between yourself and your providers so you are better informed and they are current with your individual health issues. Don't wait for an emergency.

3. With increasing patient loads and decreasing numbers of health-care providers to meet demand, digital communication technology must fill the gap to make health-care delivery more efficient, cost effective, and higher quality. This includes electronic health records, e-mail, online resources, and e-visits.

4. The e-Patient is an individual who has thought about health care and has a plan that includes evaluating the effectiveness of your health-care team. As an e-Patient, you need to be aware of your information needs. Take responsibility for your education about health matters and initiate a productive Q&A with your physician.

5. The e-Patient becomes an integral part of the team by setting goals, evaluating providers, insuring that ongoing communication is a priority and taking the lead when issues or questions arise.

Notes

1. Helen K. Reddel, et al., on behalf of the American Thoracic Society/European Respiratory Society Task Force on Asthma Control and Exacerbations, "Asthma Control and Exacerbations: Standardizing Endpoints for Clinical Asthma Trials and Clinical Practice," *American Journal of Respiratory and Critical Care Medicine*, 180 (July 2009): 59–99.
2. Wilson Pace, MD, et al., "Missing Clinical Information During Primary Care Visits," *Journal of the America Medical Association,* 293(5)(February 2, 2005):565–71.

Chapter Two

Digital Health Records Could Save Your Life

Information is the lifeblood of modern medicine. Health Information technology is destined to be its circulatory system. Without that system neither individual physicians nor health care institutions can perform at their best or deliver the highest quality care.

David Blumenthal, the National Coordinator of Health Information at the Department of Health and Human Services in the *New England Journal of Medicine*, January 21, 2010.

In the fall of 2005, Hurricane Katrina destroyed the health records of thousands of individuals in Louisiana and Mississippi. Medical officials had been warning of catastrophic medical events following a natural disaster, terrorist attack, or uncontrollable outbreak of disease. The disappearance of thousands of medical records meant that health-care providers working with these patients under emergency conditions did not have the required information at the point of care. The paper records that their physicians had kept were destroyed in the flood, and the few medical institutions that had electronic records did not back them up to a remote storage facility. With the available technology at that time, this situation should never have happened. Hopefully it will never happen again.

EHRs and PHRs

For centuries, handwritten notes made up a patient's health record and provided the basis for a treatment plan. You did not have access to this information beyond the verbal directions relayed to you by your physician. Today, your health information is in an electronic health record (EHR), which includes information that you provide to your physicians when you fill out those paper forms you are handed when you arrive at the doctor's office. Your physicians also records data based on discussions, observations, lab procedures, medications you are taking, and other information relevant to your care such as X-rays, scans, and hospitalizations. In other words, your electronic record is a complete profile of your current and past health. Many EHRs also integrate scheduling and billing functions and include decision support tools for your doctor, such as drug alerts, allergy alarms, and other treatment options that enable your doctor to care for you more effectively.

In addition to an electronic record, some of you might also have a personal health record (PHR), a computerized record that you personally create that identifies all of the providers you see, the medications you take (prescription and over-the-counter), procedures that you undergo, and your medical history. If all of the patients impacted by the Katrina floods had personal health records, their data might have been easier to retrieve when they needed to seek care. You provide all of the information that is stored in your PHR and are tasked with continually updating it. The information in both the EHR and the PHR are technically owned by you. Your EHR is generally held and maintained by your provider on your behalf, while your PHR is generated and maintained in a system that you have chosen.

Electronic health records provide your doctor with instant information, including notes from prior visits, lab tests, comments about treatments and medications, and consults with specialists. Your physician can also see the results of labs and procedures that were done years ago and pull up a history of your blood pressure or blood sugar readings, procedures, and prior tests. With an EHR, if your doctor recommends that you see a specialist, a referral can be generated right from the digital health record system to set up your appointment. Your physician may put a reminder in your EHR to follow up with the results of a test that has been ordered, or vaccines or treatments that need to be done in the future. If your doctor or a specialist you are seeing practices at a hospital that has converted to a compatible EHR system, your emergency room visits, consultations, lab test results, and inpatient records will also be in your EHR and available to all of your providers. This will make your life easier because you will not have to struggle to remember your medical history, including all current and past conditions, treatments, and medications, when you see a new physician. It will also make your life safer because there is less duplication of tests and procedures and less room for human error when all of the information is right there. If the doctor is ordering a new medication for you, those prescriptions can be sent instantly from the EHR to the pharmacy, and the system will check for adverse drug interactions with what you already take before you leave the doctor's office. If the system indicates that the medication could cause a problem for you, the doctor can order something else while you are right there.

As important as it is for your physician to have your electronic health record available during an office visit, it can be critical that your EHR is available when you go to the emergency room (ER). Imagine an eighty-two-year-old person coming to the ER with a stroke. A clot-buster drug, if administered in the first few hours, can save that person's life; however, the clot-buster is dangerous if that person is on a blood thinner, has had recent surgery, or has a history of bleeding. With a comprehensive EHR, the doctors treating that individual will know all the details that could fatally impact the treatment of the immediate critical symptoms, including the individual's health history, medications and dosages, allergies, or recent problems. The lack of this information could be catastrophic.

Although the medical world has been slow to implement electronic health records, that is changing. The American Recovery and Reinvestment Act of 2009 (ARRA) passed by congress in February 2009 includes a stimulus package that, among other things, provides significant financial incentives for doctors to implement and use electronic health records starting in 2011. By 2015, these incentive payments will be reduced. To qualify for these incentives, physicians must not only have implemented electronic records but must use their EHR in a way that is beneficial and meaningful to their patient populations. Meaningful use consists of the following elements that physicians must incorporate into their practice:

- Improve care coordination
- Reduce health-care disparities
- Engage patients and their families
- Improve population and public health
- Ensure adequate privacy and security (1)

The instant access to information enabled by an EHR results in a better information exchange between you and your doctors, as well as between your doctor and other providers who might consult on your case. All of this should improve care coordination, reduce medication errors, speed up referrals, and empower you to be more involved in your own care. By consolidating all of your health data in one place that is accessible by all of your providers and by you, the architects of the meaningful use statutes assume that these EHRs will foster better communication, engaging you and your family in managing your health.

It is a fact that your health-care provider today must cope with the enormous communication requirements that have markedly increased in the twenty-first century. The spread of digital records, e-mail, and the Internet has inundated you and your doctors with information. In the average annual visit to the doctor, numerous tests are done as a routine matter. Those tests can generate several pieces of information coming back for analysis. The analysis often leads to more tests, resulting in a lot of information to be interpreted and integrated. Years ago, the average patient could be taking two medications that had to be tracked and followed. Today many of you take multiple medications, and all need to be tracked. Neither you nor your doctor can possibly keep in your head the results of your tests, the dosages of your medications, the side effects you may experience, and the alternatives that best fit your patient profile. As a patient, you expect complete, instantaneous information, including what is wrong with you, what to do about it, who to talk to, and why it is important. To thoroughly filter all of this information, electronic records are critical. There is also evidence that electronic health records include data that enables health-care providers to better care for underserved populations and thus reduce health-care disparities. Additionally, having information electronically provides the tools that should enable health-care providers to analyze and take action on public health issues that hopefully improve health care for everyone.

Patient Benefits

You benefit from electronic health records for the following reasons:

- They generate reminders for screening tests that might otherwise be forgotten.
- Information can be shared with all of your providers and with family members who are concerned with your care.
- They provide necessary information for major surgery and procedures such as preregistration information, specific details about the procedure including how to prepare and what to expect, advice on home care, and other necessary follow-up protocols.
- They include instructions for acute and chronic conditions, such as instructions in self-monitoring, lifestyle, medications management, action plans, what to do at home, what signs of problems or improvements to look for, and when to call if symptoms develop or improvements don't occur as expected.
- They provide you with suggestions about how to prepare for scheduled visits, including questions to ask your provider and biometric instructions (e.g., the need to fast before a test).

A study conducted on behalf of the Deloitte Center for Health Solutions in 2008 with three thousand consumers indicated that three-quarters want their physician to offer online access to medical records, and one-quarter reported that they would pay for this service. Over 75 percent of individuals surveyed also said they wanted e-mail access to their physicians and online appointment scheduling, and they would pay for those services. Over 90 percent of individuals said they believed that electronic health records would improve their medical care and reduce medical error, especially in the emergency room. The majority of these individuals indicated that they wanted same-day appointments with their doctors, and they would use in-home and/or online tools to monitor their health. Why are these technologies, like e-mail, patient portals, and online visits, so slow to take hold? It is because they involve time, money, cultural barriers, education and change. (2)

Personal Health Records (PHR)

Jane, age fifty-three, lives in a rural community in South Dakota. She has been diagnosed with breast cancer, which was spotted on her annual mammogram. Her primary care physician refers her to a cancer center two hours away from her home for further screening. The doctors there decide that Jane needs surgery, followed by chemotherapy at the cancer center one hundred miles away. Prior to visiting the cancer center, Jane is instructed to collect all of her medical records, including those held by her primary care physician and gynecologist, and the X-ray films filed at her local hospital. While dealing with the trauma of a cancer diagnosis, Jane also has to navigate through the bureaucratic system to locate and copy records.

With the assistance of her PCP, Jane decides to set up a PHR that includes an extensive outline of her family's history of breast cancer, her own medical history, a list of her medications, results of labs and tests, her mammogram reports, and other scanned images. She shares the PHR with all of her doctors from the cancer center, who also provide her with the surgery and pathology reports and specifics on her treatment. Thus both her local doctors and the physicians from the cancer center are able to follow her progress and have full information on her treatment. Jane also backs up a copy of her PHR on a CD that she carries with her. At one point in her treatment, she develops a high fever and has to go to the emergency room at the local hospital. By accessing her PHR, the doctors there are able to avoid a potentially serious adverse medication reaction. Jane is an e-Patient who uses her PHR to communicate and insure her well-being.

Options for Creating a PHR

It is no exaggeration to say that a personal health record could save your life, particularly when a comprehensive electronic health record is not available. There are many ways to develop a PHR, and the method you choose is partially dependent upon what is available to you from your health-care providers or your health plan. With all of these options, except paper, you would need to have your login information with you. The following are suggestions for how to implement a personal health record.

1. You can resort to the old-fashioned handwritten synopsis of your medical heath and history on paper. This gives you a baseline

from which to work and is good for an emergency—if you remember to bring it with you. This format is not useful in a shared environment or in an emergency if the paper PHR is at home.

2. If the medical institution that you go to has a patient portal populated by data from your clinicians' electronic health record, you can superimpose your PHR and save it in the portal's database. In this model, you will have some access to your provider's electronic record data, which is connected to the existing clinical information systems. The electronic health record combined with your PHR represents a comprehensive synopsis of your medical information. Examples of this approach include My Chart at the Palo Alto Medical Clinic, PatientSite at Beth Israel Deaconess Medical Center, and My Chart at the Cleveland Clinic.

3. Your health insurer (e.g., Aetna, Blue Cross Blue Shield, or United) may provide you with the opportunity to create a PHR that will be populated with administrative claims data, such as discharge diagnoses, reimbursed medications, and lab tests ordered. The limitation of this PHR is that it is not a complete picture of your health profile, and the data could be inaccurate.

4. Many companies offer their employees personal health records that are also based upon claims data and benefit information. Typically these PHRs are hosted by an independent outsourcing partner such as Dossia, or Microsoft HealthVault. The chief problem with this approach is the question of who is going to update the information that resides in one of these storage facilities. As an e-patient, it is your responsibility to continually monitor and update your PHR, but in reality it is impractical.

5. Vendor-hosted websites such as Microsoft HealthVault, or Web MD also allow you to create, store, retrieve, and manipulate a PHR at no charge. This is as secure as an online banking site for online storage of your PHR. Examples include: www.healthvault.com, and www.webmd.com/phr.

6. You could opt to put all of your personal medical information on a USB memory stick attached to a key chain. When you want to access your health information, you plug the chip into a standard USB slot in any computer, including the systems in your health-care provider's office or the computers in the hospital emergency room. The memory stick will download the information in your PHR into the computer where a doctor anywhere in the world can view it on the screen, print it out, or transmit the information to another provider. This system does not depend upon a doctor having your electronic health record. The information on the memory stick can be encrypted so that can only be accessed with a password that you provide, thus protecting your data from unauthorized viewing.

7. There is also the PHR on a smart card, which is similar to a social security card or an ATM card. The PHR smart card includes a patient's complete health history and information on individual illnesses, as well as demographic and geographic information, insurance data, medication lists, health-care providers' names and contact information, and insurance records. You would carry your PHR smart card at all times, just like a credit card. Your primary care physician would have complete access to the medical information on the card. When you visit your PCP, the card is automatically updated with new information. Smart cards use digital signature technology with encryption and are thus more secure and private than many other forms of PHRs. In case of an emergency, the information on the smart card can be retrieved to access your medical information. However, a smart card can only be read on a compatible smart card reader, which is not available in most doctor's offices or emergency rooms. The smart card solution works best within a specific geography in a collaborative health organization or a group practice where card readers are available.

8. If you have stored your PHR in any of the online hosting sites, you can ensure that the information is always available by having a class II implantable radiofrequency transponder system implanted in your arm or leg. Although still in the experimental phase but

approved by the FDA, this implantable device, which is the size of a grain of rice, can be activated by a handheld scanner. The radio frequency identification (RFID) chip emits radio waves read by the scanner as a unique, sixteen-digit patient identification number. Your health-care provider would then use that number to access a computer database containing the medical information you previously entered and regularly update. This information includes allergies, your medication list, your medical history, the name of your primary care physician, etc. This approach presupposes you are wearing a bracelet or have some other means of identifying the implanted chip and that the facility caring for you can find the information on the Internet and use it as needed.

What Goes into a Personal Health Record?

You should include the following information in your personal health record:

1. All of the medicines you are taking, including prescription and over-the-counter medicines, dietary and herbal supplements, vitamins, and minerals. For each medicine, include the name of the doctor who prescribed it, why you are taking it, how much you take, and any special instructions.
2. A list of your allergies, including drug or food allergies.
3. Your medical history, including major health problems and chronic conditions such as asthma, hypertension, or diabetes; hospitalizations and the reasons for them; surgeries and broken bones; mental health issues including drug and alcohol issues, depression, or bipolar disorders; and illnesses such as pneumonia even if you were treated without hospitalization. Also include major health problems in your immediate family, such as heart disease, stroke, cancer, or diabetes.
4. Information that is needed in an emergency, such as whether you have a pacemaker, implanted device, or hearing or vision problems.
5. General information including identification such as a driver's license, who to call in an emergency, the name and phone number of your primary care physician, your insurance card, an organ donor card if you have one, a copy of your health care proxy, a

living will and power of attorney, your pharmacy name and phone number, and any records of insurance claims and payments.

Accurate and timely health information is a crucial element in the decision making process during a medical encounter and essential in providing you with continuity of care. Inadequate or misleading patient information can lead to medical errors, inaccurate assumptions, and increased cost. Providing your physicians with access to every detail of your medical history is difficult. Striking the balance between adequate and too much information is tricky. Your electronic health record and your personal health record have emerged as ways to address these issues and maintain that balance.

Case Studies

The following examples of how electronic records are used in key institutions illustrate why they are a critical component in providing you with safer, better quality continuous health care.

Department of Veteran Affairs, Veterans Administration Health-Care System

One of the earliest adopters of electronic health records is the Veterans Administration (VA), which in the mid-1990s embarked on an ambitious effort to improve the coordination of care by implementing an electronic health record, known as the Computerized Patient Record System or (CPRS). CPRS provides a single interface through which VA providers can update a patient's medical history, submit orders, review test results, review drug prescriptions, and perform other functions to support clinical care delivery and the promotion of wellness. The system has been implemented at all VA medical centers nationwide, and at VA outpatient clinics, nursing homes, and other sites of care. It allows any authorized person to look at patients' records, including everything from a nurse's note written during a hospital stay to the result of a blood test drawn at a clinic visit to the film of a coronary angiogram done in a cardiology lab.

CPRS allows clinicians to enter progress notes, diagnoses, and treatments each time a patient visits the doctor. Discharge summaries from the hospital, lab tests, medications, diets, radiology tests, allergies, or adverse reactions to medications and consults with other providers are all kept in this electronic health record. Built-in pop-ups remind the physician to perform certain lab tests or measurements based upon preset information. For example, if a patient has a preexisting condition such as diabetes, the system reminds the doctor to get a blood sugar level test, which can be ordered with one click. If a patient is hospitalized, portable digital wireless machines accompany the doctor or nurses right to the patient's bedside where, with patient consent, everything that is discussed becomes part of the electronic health record. VA nurses and doctors are also using bar-coded information devices that match the delivery of medications to a patient's identification bracelet worn on the wrist, a major safety initiative. Alerts have been built into the system to notify clinicians whether an order they are entering might cause a problem. Automated reminders in the EHR play a vital role in the percent of patients receiving vaccines and other screenings. With this system, flu inoculations rose to 83 percent in 2009, from 27 percent in 1995. Colon cancer screenings increased to 84 percent, from 34 percent during the same period.

Over 3.2 million veterans now have electronic health records, including many who live in rural areas of the country. These individuals benefit from one of the nation's most advanced telehealth programs in the world, which links patients and health-care providers by telephones, telephone-based data transmission, and daily monitoring of patients with chronic problems. None of this would be possible without their electronic health records.

The VA system also enables health information exchange among the more than 1,400 VA facilities, so that the medical record with the patient's history is available online to all doctors in the system, no matter where that patient shows up for treatment. Repeat MRIs, scans, blood work, or other unnecessary tests are avoided, and there is much safer medication management for the patient.

The VA's in-home monitoring program, which has about 40,000 patients enrolled, has helped reduce hospital admissions by 25 percent and length of hospital stay by 20 percent by keeping people on track and aware of changes that can be immediately addressed by on-call nurses. It is particularly vital for individuals with complex chronic illnesses, such as diabetes and heart failure. These patients use special devices provided free of charge by the VA to measure weight, heart rate, blood pressure, and other conditions. These daily results are automatically transmitted into the VA's medical record system. If the numbers exceed target levels, a nurse is notified, and a conversation between the nurse and the patient will address the problem. (3)

Kaiser Permanente

Kaiser Permanente (KP) is the largest private not-for-profit integrated health care delivery system in the United States, serving more than 8.6 million members in nine states and the District of Columbia, with headquarters in Oakland, California. The system includes Kaiser Foundation Hospitals and their subsidiaries and the Permanente Medical Groups, and it incorporates 14,000 physicians and 140,000 other staff.

KP, which champions technology-enabled care, has developed many tools that encourage its patients to communicate with their providers and manage their health. It was among the first to adopt a full-featured electronic health record. Today, all of KP's medical clinics and hospitals operate in a paperless environment. Across the system, about 14,000 physicians access electronic medical records, and many divisions have been paperless since 1998. KP doctors enter orders into exam-room computers. In the hospital, they wheel a laptop into the patient's room and record their notes as they make their rounds. KP patients can also view their information online if they wish. My Health Manager is their patient portal, which in 2009 had fifty-one million visits from patients who viewed nearly twenty-two million lab test results online and refilled approximately seven million prescriptions through the online pharmacy. My Health Manager empowers patients by providing critical time-saving features, including online appointment scheduling, twenty-four-seven online access to lab test results, eligibility and benefits information, and even their children's immunization records. KP patients also send over seven hundred thousand secure e-mails to their health-care providers in an average month. (4)

Health Information Exchange

In order to maximize the benefit of an EHR, it needs to be part of a total health solution that includes health information exchange (HIE). HIE provides the capability to electronically move clinical information among disparate information systems, such as different hospitals, while maintaining the authenticity of the information being exchanged. The benefits of sharing health information among patients, physicians, and other authorized participants in the health-care delivery chain are obvious. You often see a variety of providers to meet your health needs. For example, for treatment of a chronic condition, you could visit your primary care doctor, a specialist, a clinical laboratory, an imaging center, and a pharmacy. Each of these providers may maintain records of medical treatment, laboratory results, medications, a health history, and personal information about you that may also be needed by other providers. This information may only be available in printed format. As a result, access to your specific health data could be missing at the point of care and delay treatment. If your cardiologist is able to obtain an abnormal laboratory result electronically, this faster access could enable that doctor to perform earlier intervention for a potentially life-threatening condition.

There are also built-in safeguards with health information exchange to keep people from abusing the system. One hospital found that information obtained through its health information exchange helped its emergency department physicians ascertain that a patient who was requesting medication for pain had been in five area hospitals in seven nights seeking pain medication. Needless to say, the system allowed the professionals to stop the abuse.

In a pilot program that promises exciting opportunities for health information exchange in the future, KP and the VA have partnered to exchange health information across a Nationwide Health Information Network (NHIN). Use of this network enables clinicians from the VA and Kaiser Permanente to obtain a more comprehensive view of a patient's health across both systems. In a trial run on September 30, 2009, the VA San Diego Medical Center and Kaiser's Otay Mesa facility successfully transmitted patient data between the two hospitals via the NHIN. Since this initial launch, clinicians from the two organizations electronically, securely, and privately share authorized patient data, ensuring around-the-clock access. This is a significant achievement, since as many as 70 percent of Veterans get medical care from both the Department of Veterans Affairs and other private care providers. NHIN is a federal initiative that links health information exchanges, integrated delivery networks, pharmacies, government health facilities, labs, providers, and other stakeholders into a "network of networks." To participate in NHIN, health organizations need a gateway application that reaches across the Internet to talk to other NHIN health organizations, plus an adapter that interfaces with the organization's gateway. The VA-KP experience is a forerunner of what will become standard practice in the future.

Key Points

1. Make health care a priority in your life.
2. Talk with your providers and find out if they have an electronic health record for you. If yes, ask how you could gain access to it in an emergency. If no, ask when they envision having the technology to share your record with you and all of your providers using secure communications.
3. If you see specialists, ask your primary care physician whether or not their systems are interconnected to the specialist so your records can be shared.
4. Whether or not your physician has an electronic health record, make it a priority to create a personal health record that includes all of your medications, previous procedures, surgeries, chronic conditions, allergies, family history, and other relevant data. This PHR must contain information from your entire health history, and you must keep it up to date.
5. Be sure to monitor who has access to your PHR. Keep it in a secure environment, on your person, or in a secure site on the web.
6. Find out if there is a regional collaborative that your primary health-care group is affiliated with. Inquire whether or not you can go to any provider in the collaborative and have your information shared.
7. Become an advocate for better communication, with electronic records at the top of your agenda.

Table 1
What to Put into Your Personal Health Record

Health History	Illnesses, injuries, surgeries, chronic conditions hospitalizations, broken bones, mental Health issues: include all dates, duration, and treatment. Family related health issues.
Emergency Contact information	Health care proxy, names, phone numbers, alternate contacts
Health Insurance	Policy number, type of insurance, duration of insurance contract, co-payment information
Medications	Prescriptions including name of pharmacist; all over-the-counter medications, dietary & herbal supplements, vitamins and minerals, dosage and frequency
Allergies	Medications, foods, airborne allergies such as dust and pollen and mold, fabrics,
All of your Physicians – primary care and specialists	Name, address, phone numbers, hospital affiliations
Special situations	Permanent implants, such as joint replacements, pacemakers, special hearing or vision problems
Personal information	Living Will, Driver's license, employment history, employer, (name, address, phone), names of family members, (spouse, children, parents)

Notes

1. Center for Medicare and Medicaid Services (CMS) Meaningful Use Rules established by the to define the criteria for incentive payments for physicians who implement electronic health records, http://www.cms.gov/EMRIncentivePrograms/. Accessed November 12, 2010

2. Deloitte Center for Health Solutions, *Many U.S. Consumers Want Major Changes in Health Care Design and Delivery,* survey of 3,031 adults, Deloitte Development LLC, 2000.

3. Gary Christopherson, MD, Senior Advisor, Undersecretary for Health, Veterans Administration and Senior Fellow, Institute of Medicine; and Ross D. Fletcher, MD, Chief of Staff, VA Medical Center, Washington, D.C., in interviews with the author.

4. Homer Chin, MD, Medical Director, Clinical Information Systems, Kaiser Permanente; Howard Landa, MD, Kaiser Permanente Department of Pediatric Urology; and Eric Lederman, MD, MPH, Director of Medical Informatics, Kaiser Permanente, University of California-Davis Health Systems, in interviews with the author.

Chapter Three

Continuous Care Using E-mail, Portals, and Smartphones

Information technology has freed information from the constraints of geography and time. Information in electronic form can be made available at any place, at any time, and is not tied to a physical location. Further, software tools can make communication detailed and precise.

Joshua Meyorwitz, <u>No Sense of Place: The Impact of Electronic Media on Social Behavior</u>, Oxford University Press, 1985 p. 35.

E-mail Saves the Day

Tengis Baasanjav was born in Ulan Bator, Mongolia, with a heart condition that, if untreated, is always fatal. Doctors in Mongolia did not have the equipment and expertise to address Tengis's condition, but the baby's uncle, who was working in California, sent e-mails to cardiologists throughout the United States seeking help for his nephew. Dr. Evan Garfein, a Harvard University medical resident at Children's Hospital Boston, spotted the e-mail, and the words "pediatric cardiologist" caught his attention. He brought the case to the Chief of Cardiology, Dr. Pedro del Nido, who agreed to waive his fee and operate on Tengis. There were hurdles before surgery could take place. Dr. del Nido needed to see an echocardiogram of the baby's heart to be sure there would not be insurmountable complications. The first set of films, sent by e-mail, was inadequate for a full diagnosis. New films were forwarded to a doctor at the University of Mongolia, who was able to upload the echocardiogram to Tengis's uncle in California, who created a CD that he sent overnight to Children's Hospital. With the cooperation of several agencies helping to fund the Baasanjav family's trip to the United States and cover the hospital costs, Tengis was successfully operated on. A year later, he was walking around the family home like a normal child. (1)

Digital technology can miraculously unlock communication channels and reshape the conduct and delivery of health care to save lives and deliver better, safer medicine. Without e-mail, Tengis's story would never have reached the US doctors who cured his heart problem. On a daily basis, you are online communicating with business associates, family, and friends. You take for granted that you can find an ATM anywhere in the world to retrieve cash from your bank account. Health care does not work that way. You cannot access your health record from anywhere in the world. This limitation still exists, despite the goals set by the Institute of Medicine in 2001 when they mandated that

The health-care system should be responsible to patients at all times, twenty-four hours a day, every day, and access to care should be provided over the Internet, by telephone, and by any other means. (2)

You've Got Mail!

Conventional e-mail is the most common form of digital communication. It is inexpensive or free. It is something you use every day. However, e-mailing your doctor may not be met with a positive response. Several patient surveys indicate that people would like to communicate with doctors via e-mail, but only a tiny percent (under 10 percent) are able to do this because doctors do not use e-mail with patients. Many respondents to these surveys also reported that the use of e-mail influences their choice of a doctor. (3)

Janice lives three hours away from her doctor. She was mowing her lawn on a Saturday when she was bitten on her hand by a white-faced wasp. The hand swelled up and hurt. Janice called her PCP, who is on the staff at the Beth Israel Deaconess Medical Center in Boston (BIDMC). He told her to take a

digital photo of the bite and send it to him via e-mail. The doctor wrote back to her within a few minutes after receiving the photo and told her to ice the hand, elevate it, and watch it for twenty-four hours. If it was better, he said, do nothing; if it was worse, she should call him. She would probably have to go in to the hospital. In twenty-four hours, Janice sent another e-mail with a new photo, and sure enough, the hand looked better, the pain had subsided, and she was on the mend.

E-mail can save you from unnecessary visits to the doctor's office or the hospital in nonemergency situations. Because e-mail extends your care beyond the office visit, you can use it to ask those pressing questions that you forgot to ask, did not think about, or were embarrassed to ask when you were face-to-face with your physician. The result is a more comfortable relationship. E-mail enables you to attach photos, and both the photos and the text of your e-mail become part of your written record, providing a reference point and a history of your interactions with your providers.

Richard is an engineer with high blood pressure who checks his pressure at home daily and e-mails the readings to his doctor on a spreadsheet at the end of each week. An assistant in the office retrieves the spreadsheet and graphs the numbers, which clearly show that Richard has hypertension with a lot of variability. With this information, Richard's doctor is able to adjust his medication and get the blood pressure completely under control without the time and expense of an office or emergency room visit.

E-mail use is particularly effective in treating patients with chronic conditions who need to stay in close touch with their physicians. There are many successful examples of patients with ongoing health issues, including diabetes, hypertension, asthma, and congestive heart failure, who e-mail daily or weekly readings of their blood pressure, blood sugar, and peak flow meter to their physician's office. With this updated information, your doctor can regulate your medications, track your progress, and supply you with direct links to educational information on the web that will help you understand and manage your illness.

E-mail also spans geographic distance and enables you or your doctor to engage specialists on your behalf who might not be local. With the transmission of text and graphic images, e-mail shortens the miles between you and your PCP when you are traveling.

Deborah was on vacation in the Southwest when she injured herself climbing. She saw a local physician, who diagnosed a tendon dislocation and recommended immediate surgery. Unwilling to undergo surgery in an unfamiliar hospital, she sent an e-mail with a photo of the injury from her smartphone to her PCP, asking whether or not she could wait for surgery until she got home. Her PCP set up a consult with a local orthopedist, who reviewed what had happened and told her it was okay to wait. When Deborah arrived home two days later, everything was in place for her surgery, which was successful.

E-mail Benefits

There are many good reasons why e-mail communication is beneficial and fosters a health-care environment where continuity of care is a priority. With e-mail, your experience with your providers begins long before you walk into the office and continues long after you return home. Among the benefits of e-mail:

- E-mail takes real-time constraints out of noncritical doctor-patient communications and enables you to have an ongoing discussion, where you and your doctor exchange information asynchronously to clarify all of your issues and explain all of your concerns.
- Whether it is regulating diabetes, maintaining weight loss, overseeing your blood pressure, or handling stress, e-mail feedback between you and your providers offers the incentives needed to keep you on track.
- E-mail allows you to send graphical images so that wounds, rashes and other external injuries can be viewed, reviewed and resolved.
- E-mail provides the comfort of knowing that no matter where in the world you might be located, if you become ill, you can connect with your own physician, who will oversee your medical care and insure sure that all of your conditions and issues are being considered.

Research on weight reduction has found that people who get dieting feedback via e-mail lose more weight than people who diet without that assistance. Similar studies have shown that people who get e-mail reminders better adhere to their medication schedules than those who are not reminded, and people who receive e-mails reminding them that they have a scheduled appointment are more likely to show up. That is because e-mail provides the continuous communication and reinforcement needed for behavior modification and lapses of memory.

Privacy and Etiquette

Your medical providers may refuse to engage in e-mail communications out of concern for the privacy of your health information or the fear that you will overwhelm them with insignificant, meaningless e-mails that take time out of their busy day, time for which they are not reimbursed under the current system. Privacy of your health information cannot be guaranteed when e-mail is sent without proper encryption. Most e-mail systems have basic encryption applications built in that you should use whenever you are communicating with your providers. There are many documented cases of individuals who have sent e-mail to their physicians through company servers. Those e-mails have been intercepted, and the senders have experienced repercussions related to job advancement. In many companies, sending or receiving personal e-mail via the company server is not allowed; therefore, the company has a right to intercept and view the e-mails.

Physicians also worry about HIPAA (Health Insurance Portability and Accountability Act) regulations that outline their obligations to insure the privacy of your health information. HIPAA, which is discussed in detail in chapter 9, is legislation that defines and restricts the communication of your personal health information by your providers in order to protect the privacy of your health information. E-mail interactions are not directly addressed by HIPAA. As an e-Patient, you must be aware of privacy risks yet still advocate for e-mail use for nonemergency issues. It is also up to you to ensure that you have access to the full portfolio of communication pathways to your physicians while at the same time overseeing that your communications are secure. The guidelines below address many of the negatives associated with e-mail.

- When possible, e-mail should be sent through a secure web portal site (described on the next page) so that your privacy is protected, unless you are dealing with an issue where privacy is not a concern or a portal is not available.

- You should always encrypt your e-mail using the security settings that your e-mail system provides.
- All e-mails you send should include your full name, telephone number, and medical or hospital number so that you can be properly identified.
- Your e-mails should be concise and to the point, never trivial.
- You should always review an e-mail before sending it to avoid any ambiguities
- You should use e-mail only for standard clinical questions, nonemergencies, and in instances where you might be able to send a digital photo. Do not use it for time-sensitive requests or issues that you wish to be kept confidential.
- E-mail communications are added to your medical record.
- You should have agreed-upon expectations with your physician that e-mail communications will be answered within a reasonable span of time—twenty-four to forty-eight hours, say, not two hours or two weeks.

Patient Portals

Patient portals provide the secure communication platform needed to enable private e-mail communications. Many portals also provide you with a view into your electronic health record, and they support ancillary functions between you and your health-care provider (e.g., prescription refill requests, appointment requests, electronic case management, and lab results). Your patient portal is typically located on an Internet site designated by your provider organization, health plan, or employer, and enables you to interact and communicate with your health-care providers. Portal services are typically available on the Internet twenty-four-seven. At a minimum, patients using portals are able to review their bills, access insurance and admission forms, refill their prescriptions, schedule appointments, and look at educational tools such as videos on upcoming surgery or procedures, tip sheets on nutrition, and CDC warnings on public health threats. More robust portals offer e-messaging (e-mail) and e-visits (asynchronous conversations with your providers). You generally have to sign in to your portal each time you return. All portals are required to be HIPAA compliant.

Jack Caine, a forty-four-year-old man traveling on business, suffered a seizure and was hospitalized for several days in an institution far from his home. Using a RelayHealth portal site, his doctor was able to provide key medical information to the treating physicians and keep Jack's wife informed throughout his hospitalization. The communication between the distance doctors and the primary care physician led to a speedy recovery and much reduced stress for the family.

With a portal, your providers can send you messages such as appointment reminders, electronic statements, and notifications asking you to check your lab results. Portals have the potential to increase your involvement in your care and can be especially helpful to people with chronic conditions who use the portal to post their blood sugar, blood pressure, and other pertinent personal health information each week. An individual in the physician's office assigned to check patient information on the portal helps to insure that an irregularity will be addressed before it escalates into the need for a visit with the physician or, worse, to the emergency room. Health-care organizations are also using portals to send alerts to patients about clinical gaps in care and about scheduling exams, flu shots, and other necessary reminders.

The portal has brought a level of efficiency to patient support unattainable by the older telephone contact systems. At Memorial Sloan Kettering, where a patient portal (MYMSKCC) was launched in 2008, the most popular features among its seven thousand users are scheduling, test preparation information, and e-messaging. Patients preparing for a CT scan can find out exactly what procedures they need to follow before they come in. For those patients who use e-messaging, e-mails are routed to the appropriate administrative or nursing staff based on the message topic selected by the patient from a predefined list. With the click of a button, the message becomes part of the patient's electronic health record. (4)

On the Duke University portal, HealthView, health-care providers have shared a quarter-million test results with patients since launching in January 2008. The HealthView portal is designed to serve the roughly four hundred thousand to five hundred thousand patients using its three major hospitals and one hundred outpatient clinics. Patients, who must register to use the site, are able to access personal health information, billing and insurance information, and forms needed prior to medical visits, as well as pay their bills and schedule nonurgent appointments. Some Duke physicians are also conducting secure online consultations called e-visits. (E-visits will be discussed fully in chapter 7.) (5)

George is a seventy-two-year-old Air Force veteran who used to rush to the VA hospital in West Haven, Connecticut, as many as ten times a month for crises caused by his diabetes, multiple sclerosis, and advanced heart disease. Today, George manages much of his care at the computer, where he posts his blood sugar, heart rhythms, and blood pressure daily to the MyHealtheVet patient portal. A Veterans Affairs nurse at the nearest VA hospital checks each day to see if anything is concerning. In 2000, George was hospitalized four times. If there's a problem he can't handle by adjusting his diet or exercise, he has an e-visit with his doctor.

The MyHealtheVet portal, which has five hundred thousand registered users, provides George and other veterans with a safe, secure, and private electronic copy of their VA health information through an Internet environment. On MyHealtheVet, George can view appointments, co-pay balances, and see portions of his VA medical record. George's health history, emergency contacts, and the names and contact information for all of his providers are available to him. This health information is stored in eVault, a secure and private place where all data is encrypted. MyHealtheVet also provides George with a gateway to his veteran health benefits and services, as well as links to federal and VA benefits and resources. (6)

Smartphones

The telephone is your communication device of choice in an emergency. Ironically, health information technology had its roots in the invention of the telephone: chief among the early subscribers of telephone service were doctors and druggists. Prior to the invention of the telephone, you or someone in your family had to physically go to the doctor's office to alert the doctor of a problem. Once the telephone was commercially available, it became a reliable mode of communication, and the doctor did not necessarily have to make a house call or have you come in for a visit. The telephone is still used extensively for patient communication; however, telephone delays and telephone tag make it difficult to get the answers you need in an efficient way, given the technology now available.

Sarah is a sixty-two-year-old woman with multiple medical issues requiring her to take a daily dose of medicine that suppresses her immune system. Sara developed a painful rash on her body. She called her physician's office and reached an answering machine. The next day, Sarah called again and connected with the office receptionist, who told her that her doctor was on vacation, but the on-call doctor would be back to her by the end of the day. Although Sara stayed at home near her phone, she missed the call back. Minutes later, she could not reach anyone when she called the number left on her voice mail. On the third day, Sara called again and was scheduled for an office visit the next day—four days after her initial call. Sara was diagnosed with shingles, which can be easily controlled if caught early. Because telephone inefficiency, answering machines, and covering physicians who did not know Sara delayed her diagnosis, the shingles spread. Sara required an intensive regiment of medication and experienced a long, painful recovery.

What is wrong in this scenario is the use of an answering machine that provided no direct contact with a health-care professional and an unresponsive on-call physician who was unfamiliar with Sara's compound medical issues. If Sara had reached a medical professional at the beginning, if she had the option to send a photo of the rash via e-mail or a smartphone, she might have had a faster diagnosis and better outcome. Instead, her condition escalated, and a long recuperation resulted in repercussions and costs for her and the health-care system.

In the twenty-first century, practically every person from New York City to Hong Kong is carrying a wireless telephone or smartphone. This device is no longer just another convenient gadget. It is packed with a litany of features and has the capabilities of a computer. All smartphones run over wireless networks through radio waves or satellite transmissions and offer voice and texting. Full-feature smartphones have additional functions, such as cameras, MP3 players, downloadable games, e-mail access, and connections to the Internet. As a result, the mobile device that sits in your pocket enables you to be always online, connected, accessing and sharing information on the go. The newer smartphones, such as the iPhone, Android, Blackberry, and Palm, run on specific operating systems that enable downloading of applications similar to those available on your desktop, laptop, or smartpad. As a result, you have access to thousands of applications, including over seven thousand health, medical, and fitness applications for which you need no special training. Note that these applications may not be secure, so you must be cautious regarding what information you store on your smartphone.

The California HealthCare Foundation, a not-for-profit independent organization that supports innovation in health care and is committed to improving the way health care is delivered and financed, reported that by 2010 nearly 50 percent of Americans owned smartphones, and 80 percent of individuals had some type of mobile device. According to the study, these individuals regularly use their smartphones to seek health information online through trusted portals at institutions where they receive their care. (7)

Most people cannot part with their smartphone even for brief periods of time. Now when you call your physician's office, you are not forced to remain in one place while waiting for a return phone call. Typically, both you and your physician carry a mobile phone. If you have a particular issue that requires your medical provider to visualize your problem, you can send your doctor copies of medical photos, X-rays, MRI and CT scans, images of tumors, photos of chronic leg ulcerations, and various skin conditions directly from your phone over the wireless network. Many phones have built-in trigger systems that set off an alarm to remind you when to take your medications, in what dosage, and when you have missed a dose. You can store your health history in your phone so you do not have to struggle to remember the dates of when you might have had a surgery or a disease. Your smartphone can serve as a communication link from home monitoring devices that send data to your physician, nurse practitioner, or physician's assistant, enabling them to monitor your weight, blood pressure, blood glucose, insulin delivery, heart rate, and body temperature to better manage your chronic diseases.

It is projected that by 2015, there will be 1.4 billion people using smartphones worldwide, and they will have several million apps to choose from. Among these tools are apps intended to help you control weight, measure food portions, and adapt exercise routines. There is even an application, iStethescope, developed for physicians and used by many patients that monitors your heart rate and enables you to send that information from your phone to your doctor. Although this is in the rudimentary stages, iStethescope uses the smartphone's microphone to enhance the sound of your heart so it can be heard by your medical provider. This application will become more sophisticated and accurate, until every individual with a related cardiac issue could be continuously monitored by a provider's office for better, safer care and outcomes.

Frank suffers from sleep apnea. A Bluetooth-enabled smartphone checks Frank while he sleeps. A wireless monitor clipped to his finger or toe overnight collects data on the apnea episodes that occur during the night and sends that information to Frank's doctor over the phone. Frank and his physician analyze those episodes and decide on a treatment.

Smartphones have special features that make them well suited for your mobile twenty-first-century lifestyle. They are small, lightweight, and easy to use and handle, and they fit into your pocket. They automatically turn off when not in use. They are equipped with the ability to manage your personal information, such as a calendar, phonebook, notepad, and e-mail exchange. There are drawbacks to using a smartphone, such as the small screen, the short battery, and rampant privacy issues. Just as you do not want to send an e-mail that involves your health through the public Internet, you do not want to transmit private health information randomly through the wireless world.

With their smartphones, doctors are now plugged into evidence-based medicine, giving them the ability to apply the best available evidence gained from scientific study and discovery to their clinical decisions about how to treat you. This is a giant leap in providing you with the best possible care. At many major medical centers, doctors now carry smartphones to the bedside, where they look up the latest treatments, chart your history, and transmit that information to the hospital's central database. They can also retrieve your records from a central database, beam your information to another doctor for an easy efficient transition when a covering doctor leaves and another doctor takes over, or send a prescription directly to the pharmacy.

One unique feature of your smartphone is the ability to store an emergency contact. Let's assume that you arrive in the emergency room unconscious. If you have entered an emergency contact in your smartphone under the acronym ICE (In Case of Emergency), first responders such as paramedics, firefighters, and police officers would be able to find your contact information in the smartphone and communicate with that individual to obtain important medical information. The ICE program was conceived in 2005 after train and bus bombings in Great Britain landed hundreds of unidentified injured individuals in hospital emergency rooms. British paramedic Bob Brotchie started ICE as a grassroots movement that caught on. It has spread throughout the world's medical community. Participating in ICE could save your life. To program ICE into your cell phone:

- Access the address book feature of your cell phone.
- Enter the word "ICE".
- Enter the phone number of your husband, wife, parent, or friend—whoever would have medical information about you that would be helpful to the doctors in case of an emergency.

Anita was brought into the Montefiore Medical Center, New York City's busiest emergency room, unconscious and alone. Doctors were resuscitating her with no information about who she was or who to call until they found a cell phone in her pocket with an ICE notation in the address book. The doctors recognized the ICE acronym and located her emergency contact, who told them that Anita suffered from Type I diabetes. Having that information, the doctors were able to understand her condition and treat her appropriately. (8)

E-mail, portals, and smartphones are only as effective as their ability to empower you and your medical providers to communicate, collaborate, and expand participatory medicine to the larger community. It seems that the majority of Americans, rich and poor, well educated and not so well educated, young and old, have adapted to digital technology for business and social reasons. Over the next ten years, rapid innovation in wireless communication will provide even more features and applications to change the way that health care is delivered to you. Now is the time to adapt these tools to empower you as an e-Patient.

Overview of Consumers' Use of Health IT

Have you ever done any of these things online? BASE: ALL ADULTS (n=1,849)

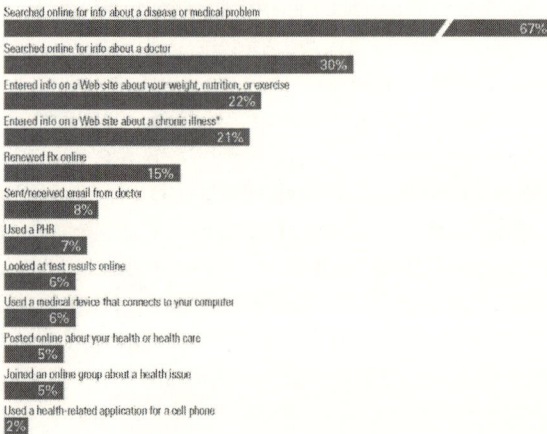

Searched online for info about a disease or medical problem — 67%
Searched online for info about a doctor — 30%
Entered info on a Web site about your weight, nutrition, or exercise — 22%
Entered info on a Web site about a chronic illness* — 21%
Renewed Rx online — 15%
Sent/received email from doctor — 8%
Used a PHR — 7%
Looked at test results online — 6%
Used a medical device that connects to your computer — 6%
Posted online about your health or health care — 5%
Joined an online group about a health issue — 5%
Used a health-related application for a cell phone — 2%

*Among those with chronic illness.
Source: Lake Research Partners, national health IT consumer survey, 2009–2010.

©2010 California HealthCare Foundation   Reprinted with permission from the California Health Foundation   4

Health IT Consumer Survey
Background
<< PREVIOUS   NEXT >>

While most adults have used the Internet to search for information on a disease or medical problem, much lower proportions have gone online to review test results or email their doctors.

Key Points

1. More is better than less when it comes to communication between patients and doctors, as long as it is done with respect and common sense. The currently available tools of communication—e-mail, smartphones, and web resources including portals—are an opportunity for you and your providers to foster the continuous care that you deserve.
2. Many doctors will not voluntarily engage in e-mail with patients, so you have to take the lead and ask for it. There must be ground rules regarding how quickly you expect your e-mails to be answered and what content is appropriate. You need to understand that e-mail should only be used for non-urgent medical matters and that the privilege of communicating via e-mail with doctors cannot be abused with too many questions or comments that waste the doctor's time.

3. Privacy of your health-care information is a continual problem, and you need to be very aware of who might read your e-mails, hear your conversations, or see your text messages. It is up to you protect yourself and to decide what information must be kept strictly confidential and when it does not matter so much.

4. The patient portal is the ideal medium where you and your physicians can exchange messages securely and asynchronously. Unfortunately for most individuals, the implementation of a portal is a physician's choice. Once it is available, however, you should make use of the portal for ongoing communications with your provider for scheduling your appointments, retrieving your lab results, and following web links posted on many portals that provide you with helpful health information resources.

5. Those who suffer from chronic illnesses such as congestive heart failure, asthma, and diabetes, can greatly benefit by using e-mail, portals, or smartphones to send daily readings to a designated individual in your provider's office so that you are closely monitored and avoid extra trips to your doctor's office or, worse, the emergency room.

6. As smartphone technology advances, messages, audio reports, and images of wounds, sores, bites, swollen limbs, etc., can be transmitted to your physicians for faster, more efficient solutions.

7. Your smartphone could even save your life if you include your emergency contact (ICE) information in your phone in case you are rushed to the emergency room unconscious and cannot identify yourself to the doctors there.

Table 2
Best Free Smart Phone-Apps

Purpose	Name	Platform
Disease Information	Epocrates Essentials Medscape	iPhone, Android, Blackberry iPhone, Android, Blackberry
Rx information and alerts	Epocrates Rx Walgreens Mobile	iPhone, Android, Blackberry iPhone, Android
Diet and Weight	Calorie Counter Spark recipes Food and Nutrition Lose it My fitness pal	Android Android Android iPhone, iPhone, Android
Fitness	Bodybuilding Runkeeper Edomodo Cardio Tracker Sports Tracker	iPhone, Android iPhone, Android iPhone, Android, Blackberry Android Nokia phones
Health Monitoring tools	Instant Heart Rate Blood Pressure Log **Blood Pressure Buddy** My Health	Android Android Android iPhone
Physician Finder	Find-A-Doc Mobile BSBSIL Doctor Finder	Android iPhone, Android Android
Symptom Checker	WebMD Symptom Checker ITriage	iPhone Android

Notes

1. Ron Winslow and Mei Fong, "Journey of the Heart: A Boston Doctor Struggled to Save a Mongolian Boy by Learning Philanthropic Medicine." *Wall Street Journal*, April 8–9, 2006. Excerpt with permission from the *Wall Street Journal* and Copyright Clearing House.

2. Institute of Medicine, "Formulating New Rules to Redesign and Improve Care," *Crossing the Quality Chasm: A New Health System for the Twenty-First Century*. National Academy of Sciences, 2001, p. 61.

3. Cheryl A. Moyer, MPH; David T. Stern, MD, PhD; Karen S. Tobias, MPH; Douglas T. Cox, MBA; Steven J. Katz, MD, MPH, "Bridging the Electronic Divide: Patient and Provider Perspectives of E-mail Communication in Primary Care," *American Journal of Managed Care* 8, No. 5, p. 427.

4. "Online Portal Connects Patients with Treatment Teams," *Center News*, Memorial Sloan Kettering Cancer Center, May 2009, http://www.mskcc.org/mskcc/html/92607.cfm, accessed July 10 2009.

5. FierceHealthIT. "Duke Launches Doctor-Patient Portal," FierceHealthIT, February 27, 2007, http://www.fiercehealth.com/duke-launches-doctor-patient-portal/2007-02-06.

6. Douglas Goldstein, story adapted from a HealtheVet case scenario, reprinted with permission from the Department of Veterans' Affairs and from the Markle Foundation.

7. Jane Sarasohn-Kahn, MA, MHSA, "How Smartphones Are Changing Health Care for Consumers and Providers," *California HealthCare Foundation*, April 2010, http://www.chcf.org.

8. Bob Brotchie, Founder, Ice for Safety, in an interview with the author. http://www.ice4safety.com.

Chapter Four

e-Patients Go to the Hospital

The best way to survive your stay in the hospital is quite obviously never to end up there in the first place.

Evan Scott Levin, MD, <u>What Your Doctor Won't (or Can't) Tell You</u>, G.P. Putnam & Sons New York, 2004.

Evolution of the Hospital

American hospitals have had an interesting history. The first hospitals were makeshift structures used by the military during the colonial era and the Revolutionary War or as quarantine hospitals during epidemics. By the early nineteenth century, sick, poor individuals were treated at alms houses, many of which ultimately became tax-supported municipal hospitals run by local governments. During that era, wealthy individuals were tended at home. Going to the hospital was considered a last resort appropriate only for those who had no other choice.

The first permanent institutions for the general care of the sick were organized in Northeastern cities in the eighteenth and early nineteenth centuries and included Pennsylvania Hospital in 1751, New York Hospital in 1771, and Massachusetts General Hospital in 1821. During the antebellum era (pre–Civil War), the industry saw the growth of many similar general-care hospitals and some specialty hospitals, including asylums or mental hospitals, "lying-in" hospitals associated with foundling homes (unwanted children), and hospitals for the care and treatment of the blind. The link between poverty and hospitalization remained strong during that period.

After the Civil War, the number of hospitals increased dramatically, due not so much to medical advances but to surging immigration and rapid urbanization. By 1900, there were approximately 1,400 hospitals, mostly organized by religious groups or local governments. These municipal hospitals were typically larger than the others and were supported by public funds and managed by public authorities. Many developed reputations for grim conditions. They relied on patient payments to remain financially sound. Finally, there were some private hospitals that derived most of their financial support from philanthropists, supplemented by public funding. As expanding hospital populations outpaced traditional sources of funding, patients at all of these facilities increasingly paid out-of-pocket for their hospital treatment. This helped remove the stigma of hospitalization as a last resort for paupers.

Hospital growth continued unabated in the early twentieth century, with the number soaring to more than six thousand by the mid-1920s. The hospital's image as a charity institution faded, and many hospitals advertised comfortable private rooms to attract patients. The nineteenth-century institutions had mainly treated individuals with severe chronic conditions. These twentieth-century hospitals typically welcomed the acutely ill as well as surgical and obstetrical cases. The number of women delivering their babies in hospitals also increased, especially after 1914, when a sedative to induce "twilight sleeps" that offered the promise of painless childbirth was introduced. This proved crucial to the emergence of the modern hospital. During that early twentieth century era, nursing schools and medical schools evolved to provide a steady supply of student nurses and medical students to staff wards. Institutional and professional groups formed, including the American Hospital Association and the American College of Surgeons, whose mission was the modernization of all aspects of hospital life, from record-keeping to laundry practices. By the end of the 1920s, deliveries and abortions, adenoidectomies, appendectomies, tonsillectomies, and the treatment of accident victims accounted for 60 percent of hospital admissions. By 1935, a third of Americans were born in and died in a hospital, but regional and class differences still persisted.

In an ironic twist, high fees charged for hospital care increasingly excluded the hospitals' traditional patients, the poor.

Even before World War II, proposals for compulsory national health insurance engendered powerful discussions but did not become law. Meanwhile, voluntary hospital insurance plans, such as Blue Cross, emerged and flourished. The 1946 Hill-Burton Act provided substantial funding through federal grants to states for hospital construction. The states in turn allocated the available money to their various municipalities, creating a network of local hospitals with the intention of achieving 4.5 beds per 1,000 people. Facilities that received Hill-Burton funding had to adhere to several requirements that would shape the hospital environment for years to come:

- They were not allowed to discriminate based on race, color, national origin, or creed, though separate but equal facilities in the same area were allowed.
- Facilities that received funding were required, for a twenty-year period, to provide a "reasonable volume" of free care each year for those residents in the facility's area who needed care but could not afford to pay.
- The federal money was also only provided in cases where the state and local municipality were able to match the federal grant or loan.(1)

Financial issues continued to be central to hospital development. In 1965, Medicare and Medicaid programs provided hospitals with reimbursement for care of the elderly and the poor, which shaped the payment system we have today. In the 1970s and 1980s, as hospital costs climbed, many voluntary hospitals merged, creating regional and national chains. The number of for-profit hospitals rose from 414 in 1977 to 797 in 1997. The 1990s found America's hospitals in a state of financial crisis, aggravated by insurance pressures. As a result, many hospitals shortened patient stays, performed more surgeries on an ambulatory basis, contracted out medical testing, and shifted recuperating patients to less-expensive venues. These changes not only impacted the economics of running the hospital but resulted in raising the quality of care so that there were fewer hospital acquired infections. Most of these health-care policies remain in effect today.

How Do You Choose a Hospital?

There are times when you have an emergency and are taken to the closest hospital emergency room. Although in this situation you do not choose where you are going, once your emergency is addressed, you have the option of being transferred to the hospital of your choice. The actual transfer usually will take place at your personal expense. There are also instances when you know in advance that you are going to the hospital. You want to think carefully about where you are going, who is going to take care of you, and what criteria are important in making your choice. Here are some tips to help you.

1. **Are you covered?**
   One of the primary factors in choosing a hospital is whether or not your hospital expenses will be covered by your health plan. Hospitalizations can run into several thousand dollars per day, and you need to go to a facility where most of those charges do not come out of your pocket.

2. **Is your doctor on staff?**
   If your primary care doctor is not on staff, and you and your doctor agree a particular hospital is the best place to address your particular needs, be sure your doctor can refer you to someone at that hospital who will handle your overall care.

3. **What type hospital best serves your needs?**
   There are several types of hospitals, and they serve different populations and health-care issues:
   - **General hospitals and community/municipal hospitals** deal with a broad range of medical conditions and can adequately address most common illnesses and surgeries. Your local hospital is often more convenient for you and is the place where you will see your primary care physician.
   - **Specialized care hospitals** address specific diseases or conditions (e.g., cancer centers, children's hospitals, mental health hospitals, and orthopedic centers). They could be the best option if you have a condition that requires the care of physician specialists who are experienced in the unique issues of your particular illness.

- **Teaching hospitals,** affiliated with medical schools, are generally larger than community hospitals and handle more comprehensive care issues. At a teaching hospital, you will be seen by medical students, interns, and residents as well as your own doctors. Your in-hospital care could be handled mainly by a hospitalist (a doctor who practices only in the hospital and is familiar with some of the special situations that arise with inpatients) rather than your regular doctor. There are reasons why you might choose your local hospital versus a teaching hospital. The quality of care at a community hospital, especially for routine procedures and surgeries, will likely be as good as it will be at a teaching hospital and will cost less money. On the other hand, if you are in the hospital for a diagnosis that is complicated and rare, the cutting-edge research and technologies of the teaching hospital may be what is needed to offer you the best possible care available.
- **For-profit hospital** charges are typically higher than the not-for-profit community hospitals for similar procedures. Studies show that there is a higher incidence of adverse events at for-profit hospitals. If you choose a for-profit hospital, you need to investigate the particular institution closely before making a decision. Information that rates all hospitals is available on the web and listed in this chapter.(2)

4. **Staff Questions**
    You want a hospital that is adequately staffed so that you will get the care you need to get well. Questions to investigate about the staff include:
- How many registered nurses (RNs) are on staff? What is the nurse-to-patient ratio? One nurse can effectively care for three to six patients except in the ICU, where the ratio should be one nurse to every one or two patients.
- Who is the infection control practitioner? The hospital may not have someone with that specific title, but there should be an individual in charge of coordinating infection control, since as many as 5 percent of patients in the United States pick up a hospital-acquired illness during their stay.

- Who is the ombudsman? Ombudsmen work as go-betweens for patients and hospitals to handle complaints. Be sure to investigate who is charged with this responsibility.
- How many social workers are on staff? Social workers assist patients in dealing with everything except actual medical issues. This includes emotional, social, clinical, and financial issues, as well as post-hospitalization care plans.

5. **What do people say about the hospital?**
    You need to talk with family and friends about the hospital you are choosing. Ask them about their experience and success in treating their health problem. You can also go online and search for articles, ratings, and blogs about the hospital you are considering. You want to know how many similar cases are seen there each year and the results. If you are having surgery, try to choose a hospital and a doctor that does your specific surgery frequently. If you are particular about the amenities that the hospital offers, check to see if they have what you are looking for. Many hospitals today offer private rooms, massage therapy, and beauty treatments for a fee. If this is important to you, put that into the equation.

6. **Accreditation**
    Be sure the hospital is accredited by the Joint Commission that rates hospitals. Go to: www.jointcommission.org/accreditation/hospitals.aspx.

    There are also several websites that you where you can check on hospital standings.

    www.hospitalcompare.hhs.gov

Hospital Compare was created through the efforts of the Centers for Medicare and Medicaid Services (CMS), the Department of Health and Human Services, and other members of the Hospital Quality Alliance: Improving Care through Information (HQA). At this site, you will find information on how well hospitals care for patients with certain medical conditions or surgical procedures and the results of patient surveys about the quality of care they received during a recent hospital stay.

www.consumerreports.org/health/doctors/hospital-ratings.htm

The Consumer Reports Patient Ratings are based on survey responses from millions of patients and include how well doctors communicate, how attentive the hospital staff is, and more. The responses are sorted by state and location and include ratings based on how reliably a hospital performs recommended steps before and after surgery to prevent infections and how often patients acquire bloodstream infections while in an intensive-care unit. Hospitals are also compared on how aggressively or conservatively they treat serious chronic medical conditions.

www.qualitycheck.org

This is a website of the Joint Commission on Accreditation of Healthcare Organizations and provides the most comprehensive listing of health-care organizations available.

www.healthgrades.com

Health Grades rates both doctors and hospitals. In fact, you are able to search information by state and city and then by specialty. On this site, you can find ratings on patient survival immediately after hospitalization and on survival six months after a hospital stay. You can also search for hospitals by the awards they received. Information for these ratings is collected from the Centers for Medicare and Medicaid and from the Leapfrog Group, which seeks to reduce preventable medical mistakes and improve the quality and affordability of health care.

7. **Recovery Services**
   With all hospitalizations, there is going to be a recovery period. It could be a combination of hospital recovery care, rehabilitation care, and at-home care. Before you go into the hospital, you need to plan for your recovery period. Seek assistance from hospital staff in finding the right rehabilitation program that will enhance your recovery. Arrange for help at home. Be sure that the hospital has adequate resources to help you with this issue.

What Happens in the Hospital?

Evelyn, a seventy-five year old woman who suffered from rheumatoid arthritis and congestive heart failure, fell and fractured her hip. She called 911 and was rushed to the community hospital, where she underwent surgery. After three days, Evelyn was sent to a rehabilitation facility. During her first couple of days there, she made progress and worked with a physical therapist to begin to walk again. On the third day, however, she became weak and tired. Because she complained of pain, her medication dosage was increased by the nurses. The fourth day, Evelyn became unresponsive and confused and could not get out of bed. Family members questioned the staff and asked to have her seen by a physician. They were told that there were no doctors coming in to check the patients until the end of the week (five days later). The family took action, called their internist at the Massachusetts General Hospital (MGH), and with Evelyn's permission, had her transferred. By the time she arrived at the ER at MGH, she was nearly comatose, unresponsive, and hallucinating. The doctors changed and adjusted her medications, and over a two-week period, her physical condition improved and her mental acuity returned. She went to a different rehab hospital to continue the physical therapy that would help the hip heal and where she was taught to walk again. Evelyn lived on for many years after that incident, but had the family not taken action and changed her venue, the medications that were causing adverse reactions could have killed her.

In another example of medical error, three hospitalized babies died after receiving an overdose of the same drug. In the three different occurrences, nurses mistakenly administered a concentration of the medication heparin a thousand times higher than intended, giving these babies a dose with a concentration of ten thousand units per milliliter instead of the correct dosage of ten units per milliliter. (3)

These examples offer vivid illustrations of how easily medication overdose or confusion about medications and dosages can have horrific results. Since these events, drug manufacturers have repackaged many medications and include large "red alert" symbols on the more concentrated doses. Through education and marketing, nurses and doctors have become more aware of drug-drug interactions and the need to closely monitor patients, particularly the elderly. Nevertheless, medication errors are still among the

51

most common medical errors, harming at least 1.5 million people annually, according to the Institute of Medicine of the National Academies. The extra medical costs of treating drug-related injuries occurring in hospitals alone conservatively amount to $3.5 billion a year. This estimate does not take into account lost wages and productivity or additional health issues. Many hospitals now have bar coding that checks a medication against a patient record and again directly with the patient's ID bracelet to be sure the individual is being given the right medication in the right dosage at the right time. In October 2008, the Department of Health and Human Services (HHS) reported that of nearly one million Medicare beneficiaries discharged from hospitals in that month, about one in seven experienced an adverse event and was harmed. These events include infections, falls, and medication errors. The same study showed that over 44 percent of the adverse events could have been prevented with appropriate attention. (4)

Computer physician order entry (CPOE), where physicians enter their orders directly into a computer to replace handwritten order sheets and prescription pads, helps to avoid some of these medication errors. The built-in decision support capabilities included in most CPOE systems trigger mechanisms warning of an allergy or drug-drug interaction. At hospitals where CPOE systems are in place, medications come to the patient's bedside faster, which can shorten the length of stay. If there is bar coding, medication errors are even more reduced.

A seventy-one year old man with congestive heart failure was admitted to the hospital. He did not have a preadmission diagnosis of diabetes. In the emergency room, he had a routine blood test and his blood sugar was elevated. At 11:30 p.m., the nurse notified the covering intern, who ordered an insulin dosage to be given to him. At 1:10 a.m., his blood sugar was checked once again by a different nurse and was elevated even more. The intern ordered more insulin. At 3:00 a.m., another blood test was taken, and the intern ordered more insulin. At 11:00 the next morning, a different covering intern was notified that this man's blood sugar level continued to rise, and eight units of insulin were given intravenously. At 3:40 p.m., the patient was unresponsive, and another blood check revealed a low blood sugar. Later it was discovered that many of the blood specimens had been drawn incorrectly, resulting in a false reading. Fortunately, the patient revived with no lasting harm.

One of the most common causes of in-hospital error happens when new shifts of doctors and nurses are assigned to cover a patient, and full information, including the patient's history and a full assessment of the patient's problems, is not communicated at the point of care. As the above case illustrates, when the medical staff do not have the right information, it is a set-up for medical error. As an e-Patient in the hospital, as long as you are conscious, you should check each medication you are given before it is administered. Ask your nurse about every pill and what is in the intravenous medication attached to your arm. If you do not recognize the medication or cannot get a satisfactory explanation, refuse it until you talk with your doctor. That is your right.

Another issue to be aware of when hospitalized is the prevalence of hospital infection. Hospital-acquired infections have been rising every year. Basic standards for hand hygiene, sterile handling of equipment, and proper use of antibiotics can go a long way in reducing these hospital borne infections. You have to keep your ears and eyes open and think about the hygiene around you. Most hospitals have instituted a policy of hand-washing and have special soap dispensers just outside or right inside patient rooms and on all floors. If you do not see your doctor or nurse washing their hands before they examine you, politely insist that they comply with this rule. Make sure that you wash your hands frequently as well, since you come into contact with the germs latent in the hospital equipment, along the corridors, and on hospital personnel. You are the first line of defense.

Beginning in October 2012, Medicare payments to hospitals will be tied to how well they protect patients from these infections and perform on other patient safety issues. A reporting system adopted by the HHS will enable you to find out how various hospitals perform in relation to similar institutions when it comes to preventing certain infections.

This ruling also addresses the prevalence of in-hospital patient falls. Accidental falls are among the most common safety incidents affecting hospital inpatients and home-care residents. You need to be diligent about asking for help when you have to get out of bed. You may feel the nurses are really busy and you do not want to disturb them, but you do not want to risk a fall that results in broken bones or worse. When you have been ill and are recuperating, you are weaker than normal. With the medications you take in the hospital, you could easily get dizzy and fall. You need to speak up and request help until you are well enough to move about on your own. If that help is not given willingly, speak with the supervisor on the floor or speak to the social worker assigned to your care.

Technology Improves Patient Care

When the doctors at the VA make rounds, they do so with a laptop computer on a portable cart, where they enter notes right at the patient's bedside. The doctors use smartphones that have a database of the patient's bar-coded information, and they match that to the identification barcode on the patient's wristband. All medications also have their own bar-coded identification. Before medicating a patient, a nurse or staff member laser scans three barcodes: the one in the computer, the one on the medication, and the one on the patient's wrist. The scans are entered into the computer. Within seconds, software verifies that medication is for that individual and the dosage is correct. The program screens for half a dozen potential problems, such as drug interactions. If everything checks out, the software simply records the event, preserving the information in an electronic record. The system flashes an immediate warning if anything is out of order. The system makes it very hard to give the patient the wrong medication. The VA has experienced a significant reduction in medication errors.

There is no question that digital communication technology has revolutionized the way doctors, nurses, and other professional staff are able to communicate with each other and with you to provide better, safer care. It will only get better in the future. Today, portable tele-video stations placed at patient's bedside enable specialists who have similar systems in their home to consult twenty-four-seven with attending physicians, residents, and interns on complex cases. In some hospitals, robotic workstations with screens and cameras are visiting patients and communicating visual information and data back to the doctor in his or her office. Smartphones enable doctors to hook into the hospital's larger computer systems to access a patient's electronic record at the bedside and get immediate feedback from the cardiac monitors or from labs while they are in their office or en route to see you in the hospital. These same doctors can engage in an instant telephone consultation with their colleagues to discuss your care. Several studies indicate that over 80 percent of doctors now use smartphones. Patients too are using their smartphones to find a trauma center or a hospital when they are on the move.

A Visit to the Emergency Room (ER)

The fast response and critical care nature of the emergency room requires your special attention because the potential for error is high. In the ER, the staff is working under extremely stressful conditions, and the complexity of the issues they confront is daunting. Last year, there were nearly 118 million visits to emergency rooms in US hospitals. Over 12 percent resulted in hospital admissions; nearly 40 percent were injury related, and nearly 2 percent resulted in a transfer to another hospital. The number of ERs across the country has decreased while the number of visits has increased. One-fifth of the civilian non-institutionalized population had at least one ER visit in 2007. As a result, ERs are experiencing higher patient volume and overcrowding. When you are in the ER, you will wait a longer time to be treated for a minor issue while the more serious cases are triaged ahead of you. That is because ERs provide critical, often life-saving, treatment, which is their primary purpose. (5)

As an e-Patient in the ER, you need to be completely aware of what treatment you are receiving and who is taking care of you, as the staff with its frenetic pace could be prone to making errors. Always try to go to the ER with an advocate (friend or family member). Keep an emergency (ICE) contact in your cell phone. You need to communicate fully all of the information about your medications, allergies, chronic conditions, and special issues, or be sure that your advocate can do this for you so that the providers attending to you have complete information to treat you without mishap.

Nicholas had been experiencing chest pains for ten minutes when his wife made the call to 911. Within minutes, an ambulance arrived and swiftly transported him to his local municipal hospital, where a physician was waiting in the ER to examine him and provide immediate treatment. The Emergency Medical Services squad kept in touch with the ER team using a two-way phone connection. After hooking Nicholas up to the appropriate monitors, taking blood, and talking with him about his symptoms, the on-call cardiologist arrived. Depending on the diagnosis, Nicholas could be sent to the Chest Pain Center for monitoring, to the cardiac catheterization lab, to surgery, be admitted for further evaluation, or be discharged and referred for follow-up care. His wife was allowed to remain at his side during the entire time. Because of the urgent nature of his condition, he was triaged into immediate care services and experienced no wait to be seen. The decision was made to send Nicholas directly to the cardiac catheterization lab.

Several hospitals are using a digital dashboards in the ER to track and monitor patients. When patients are admitted, their demographic information, including medications, tests, procedures, and lab results, populate the dashboard. The system provides a real-time view of what is going in the ER at any particular time, showing updates on each patient. The results are stored, and the dashboard sends alerts to the staff indicating where patients are located and what is happening with them. Patients are identified by their initials to protect privacy, and there are indicators to shows how long a patient has been waiting.

Case Study: The Dashboard at BIDMC

At the Beth Israel Deaconess Hospital in Boston, several staff members got together to create a special workflow system similar to that used by airport traffic control. They use computer monitors to tell them which patients are coming in, who is languishing in a delay pattern, and where all patients are located. The system includes patient admitting information and a full discharge summary, all medication information, and other relevant medical history that is normally on a paper chart. A wireless phone network enables the attending physicians, interns, and residents to communicate with physicians outside the hospital and keeps everyone on the same page in terms of information about the patients. If a patient comes in unconscious but has a driver's license, the staff can access pharmacy information and patient treatment records from affiliated hospitals. A barcode tag system that scans the patient's armband and the tag on hospital equipment enables staff to identify where their equipment is being used and triage it to the most vital cases. Each doctor carries a phone connected to an internal network, an extension of the hospital system, so the doctors can communicate with one another immediately. Thus, physicians can continue their patient care activities and do not have to waste time waiting by a phone for a call back. On the wireless phone system, there is a special number that rings to a senior physician and allows clinicians at other area hospitals direct access for assistance in transferring their most challenging cases. At BIDMC, all prescriptions are electronically stored, so if the emergency room visitor is a patient of the hospital, their medication records are immediately accessible. The dashboard helps the staff make decisions based on the status of individual patients and patient flow and provides information on trends in the ER that can help identify problems. The system has increased efficiency and decreased patient frustration and wait time. (6)

Leaving the Hospital

When you are about to be released from the hospital, you must be sure you go through a checklist with your nurse regarding your follow-up and treatment instructions. The checklist should include these questions:

- Who is your discharge planner? How do you contact that individual if you need information after you are released?
- What medications should you be taking, including dosages, time to take the medication, and how to get refills if needed?
- Be sure to understand changes to your previous medication regimen.
- When are you to see the doctor for a follow up visit?
- Are all IV catheters tubes and patches removed? You do not want to have to return to have those taken out.
- Do you need to talk with someone from the admitting office about any outstanding paperwork, health insurance, or billing questions?
- Who is lining up resources for you to have physical therapy, occupational therapy, or other types of rehabilitation therapy that you might need?

Key Points

1. Although we would like to think of hospitals as safe havens of care, this is not always the case. It is incumbent upon you to be diligent in your hospital choice and aware of the risks and dangers when you are a patient in the hospital.
2. If you are too sick to advocate for yourself, you must have someone with you who can assume that responsibility. That person must be

willing to ask tough questions and be assertive if something seems amiss. If you do not have a family member or personal friend to be your advocate, ask the hospital to supply a social worker to work with you.

3. Be sure to ask your doctors what medications are prescribed for you, at what dose, and how often you are to take the medication. Ask the nurses about your medications every time that they are brought to you, or have your advocate do that if you are too ill. This will help to ensure that you are receiving the right drug, in the right dose, at the right time.

4. Inquire about drug interactions. Most hospitals have computerized alert systems. Ask your nurses and doctors if there are any warnings about the combinations of drugs you are receiving.

5. Note when you are given a drug if you are feeling any different—dizzy, lightheaded, nauseous, etc. Don't assume that it is part of being sick. Convey your physical feelings immediately to your nurse, who can double check the drug and call the doctor if you are having a bad reaction.

6. Avoid falls. Do not get out of bed without assistance until you are totally certain that you are able to do so. Wear footwear with rubber soles to prevent slipping. Be sure to report any spills or objects that are on the floor. Use all bars and handles made available to you for balance.

7. Keep personal items, such as medications, drinks, books, the TV remote, and especially the call button near you at all times so that you do not have to get out of bed.

8. Do not hesitate to use the call button if you have a genuine need. Make sure that you have adequate light to see. If you wear glasses, keep them within reach.

9. If you are on medications that cause you to use the bathroom frequently, ask the nursing staff to schedule time to help accompany you.

10. Observe whether your nurses, doctors, other hospital workers, and visitors use the hand wash dispenser before they come in to see you. Ask everyone coming into your room to wash their hands if they fail to do so.

11. Be sure you understand a proposed surgery. Know exactly what will occur during the operation and who will attend to your care

after the surgery, both while you are in the hospital and while you are in rehabilitation and when you get home. Be sure that your anesthesiologist is aware of any problems, allergies, or bad reactions you may have had in prior surgeries or procedures where anesthesia was administered. Be clear about follow-up care when you leave the hospital.

12. When you are being discharged, make sure you get detailed instructions about your medications, diet, and exercise. Find out what symptoms might be worrisome and ask for a number to call if anything goes wrong. If you will need home care services, a skilled nursing facility, physical therapy, or occupational therapy, get a list of referrals and set up dates for the visits ahead of time. Make sure you leave with a plan for your follow-up care. Be sure you understand what signs and symptoms you should watch out for and what you should do if you have them.

Notes

1. Hill-Burton Program, *Hill-Burton Free and Reduced Cost Healthcare* (US Department of Health and Human Services Health Resources and Service Administration, July 2010). http://www.hrsa.gov/hillburton/default.htm.
2. Gordon Schiff, "Fatal Distraction Finance vs. Vigilance in Our Nation's Hospitals," *Journal of General Internal Medicine*, April 15, 2000, pp. 269–270. PMCID: PMC 1495441. http://www.ncbi/nlm/nih.gov/pmc/132358/.
3. Tom Davis, "Deaths of Three Babies in Indiana Spotlight Medication Mix-Ups," *Boston Globe*, Associated Press, September 23, 2006.
4. Office of News and Public Information, National Academy of Sciences, July 2006. http://www.nationalacademies.org/opinnews/newsitem.aspx.
5. National Hospital Ambulatory Medical Care Survey, 2007 Emergency Department Summary.Tables 1, 4, 10, 12, 21. http://www.cdc.gov/nchs/ahcd.htm.
6. Larry A. Nathanson, MD, Director of Emergency Medicine Informatics, the Beth Israel Deaconess Medical Center, in an interview with the author.

Chapter Five

Patient Safety: How to Ensure Your Well-Being

Mistakes are a fact of life. It is the response to error that counts.

Nikki Giovanni, 1943, African–American poet, essayist, author, and editor William Morris, <u>Black Feeling, Black Talk, Black Judgment</u>, 1970

Josie, an eighteen-month-old baby girl, was admitted to a prestigious East Coast hospital after suffering burns when she climbed into a hot bath. Her mother kept a vigil at her bedside. While in the hospital, Josie became severely dehydrated. Her mother heard the doctor tell the staff that Josie was not to receive any more medication. Shortly thereafter, a nurse came in with more pain medication for Josie. The mother questioned the nurse, who said the orders had been changed. Fifteen minutes later, Josie's heart stopped. She had suffered cardiac arrest as a result of dehydration caused by the medication. Two days later, Josie was taken off life support, and she died in her mother's arms. Her death was preventable. (1)

Medical errors happen far more often than need be. At the beginning of 2001, the Institute of Medicine (IOM) of the National Academies reported to the American public that tens of thousands of deaths occur each year due to medical errors. "At least 44,000 and as many as 98,000 Americans die from medical errors that occur in hospitals each year." (2) "These medical errors kill more people per year than breast cancer, AIDS, or motor vehicle accidents." (3) "These numbers are more than the number of Americans who died in the Korean and Vietnam wars combined, as reported by official Pentagon sources." (4)

Although is it true that human beings, including medical professionals, make mistakes, studies conducted by the National Institute of Health have shown that as many as 40 percent of these mistakes are preventable.

Patient Safety: A Hallmark of Excellent Care

Patient safety problems of all types happen during the course of receiving health care. Many are preventable; some are inexcusable; all are unwarranted. These errors are made by good but fallible people working with imperfect systems. Today's physicians and nurses have more potent medications to administer to patients, more complex and technologically advanced equipment to diagnose disease and deliver treatment, and much more information to process. These innovations create opportunities for error because they are not always accompanied by the robust infrastructure needed to manage each and every patient. There are many specific causes of medical errors, which account for one-half of all the medical costs annually in the United States. They include illegible writing in medical records, inaccessibility of records, inability to automatically check for allergy and drug interactions, and missing information about a patient at the point of care. Additionally, many Americans do not receive appropriate care for chronic illnesses like diabetes and hypertension, which leads to thousands of preventable second heart attacks, kidney failures, painful and debilitating fractures, and other serious but sometimes irreversible conditions.

Specific examples of medical errors include:
- Adverse drug events
- Transfusion errors
- Wrong-site surgery
- Surgical injuries (such as leaving foreign bodies inside the patient)
- Preventable suicides
- Restraint-related injuries or deaths
- Hospital-acquired or other treatment-related infections
- Falls

- Burns
- Pressure ulcers
- Mistaken identity
- Poor care in rehab facilities
- Order entry errors
- Diagnostic errors

On July 25, 2005, President George H. W. Bush signed Public Law (PL) 109-41, the Patient Safety and Quality Improvement Act of 2005. This law was a response to the Institute of Medicine report "To Err Is Human," which outlined the preponderance of medical errors experienced by the patient population at the beginning of this century. This report set standards of quality, performance, and patient safety that health-care institutions are now required to meet. The bill includes provisions for disclosure of medical errors. It also outlines a process that certifies which patient safety organizations are authorized to maintain data about medical error and oversee the quality and safety performance of all US health-care institutions. These standards provide a safety net for everyone.

Among the key provisions of the law are:
- The establishment of a center for patient safety within the Agency for Healthcare Research and Quality (AHRQ).
- The establishment of a nationwide mandatory reporting system by state
- Performance standards and expectations for health-care organizations
- A mandate for the FDA to develop standards for the safe packaging of medications and the naming of drugs so the names do not confuse and overlap
- Provisions for the legal protection of patient safety data so that health-care providers are encouraged to voluntarily report this incidents to appropriate public services organizations

What You Can Do to Protect Yourself and Your Family

There are actions that you can take to insure the safety of your care:

1. General Health Oversight

- **Develop your PHR (detailed in chapter 2).** You must have a continuous care record that stays with you from birth to death. You can make this record available to all of your health-care providers anywhere in the world. This record will provide you and your health-care team with full access to the right information and resources to address diseases and conditions that you may face. It is the only way to insure that all of the providers you encounter have your complete information.
- **Find a health-care gatekeeper.** You need to have a primary care provider who is fully aware of your medical conditions and who can coordinate your care with members of your health team, and who is available to answer all of your personal health concerns.
- **Make sure you have full access to care.** This includes the flexibility to get a second opinion when an initial diagnosis or treatment plan does not seem quite right, the ability to have a lab test or go to a hospital when you feel there is a valid need, the capability to access to your medical record so procedures and tests are not duplicated, and the availability of results.
- **Do not assume anything!** Make sure that all health professionals involved in your care have all the important health information about you.
- **Ask questions**. If you have a test, be sure to get the results and have the results explained to you. Don't assume that if you hear nothing that everything is okay.
- **Learn about your conditions and treatment** by asking questions and checking reliable Internet sources. (See chapter 8 for web resources.)

2. Your Visit with the Doctor

- Research the physicians in your community or those suggested by your health plan and select a doctor that you will be comfortable with. (See chapter 8 for websites that evaluate doctors.)
- Schedule an appointment with your doctor. Don't just assume that you can walk in and see your physician. If you need a referral, be sure to get one well in advance of the appointment.
- Be sure to bring every piece of information that would be helpful to your physician. This includes all previous health records, X-rays and lab reports, a written, comprehensive list of your medications, your full medical history, your health insurance card, and a list of questions.
- Arrive early, at least fifteen minutes before the appointment. Sometimes there are forms to fill out before you see the doctor.
- Make sure you and the doctor stick to the purpose of the visit and you do not wander off into discussions about issues that are not relevant to the reason you are there. Develop a plan with your physician about addressing other issues after the visit.
- Request handouts or web references for more in-depth information about your treatment or conditions.
- Be sure that you do all the necessary follow-up after your visit. Review the information, recommendations, and medications; make sure you understand exactly what the instructions are; take the full course of medication prescribed; follow-up with the doctor; and be sure that you personally get the results of any tests or address any further issues that arise.
- If surgery or a procedure is recommended, be sure you understand why the procedure is needed, what the risks are, what the success rate for the surgery is, who you can consult for a second opinion, what post-surgical issues you will face including pain management, the expected time for recovery, potential risks and side effects, short—or long-term disabilities, and how frequently that surgery is performed at the recommended hospital. Also check into what type of anesthesia will be used. Be sure to have a family member or friend available to advocate for you when you are in the hospital and unable to advocate for yourself.

3. Understanding your Rights

- You have the right to fire your physicians if you do not like the way they treat you, if you do not trust them, or if you do not believe they are providing you with the best possible care. You might be limited to choosing a physician within your health plan if you do not want to pay exorbitant rates for your care, but you have the right to make a change.
- Take an active interest in your care and treatment. Ask any question of your physician that you feel is important to you. Do not get hung up on the idea that it is a "stupid" question. You have the right to ask and to receive an honest answer.
- Be told about alternative courses of treatment, even if your health insurance may not cover them or you may not be able to afford them. If you find that your physician is saying things like, "Well, there is another option, but you probably can't afford it," make it clear that you want to hear about all of the options for treatment.
- You have the right to refuse to consent for any procedure or treatment. If you refuse consent, you may be asked to read and sign a form indicating that refusal.
- You have the right to leave a hospital or care facility against medical advice. You will likely have to sign a waiver indicating that you are doing so of your own free will and against the recommendations of your medical providers.
- If you participate in a medical or drug trial, you have the right to ask specific questions regarding the purpose of the trial, the potential risks of the trial, the benefits which you may receive, payments to which you may be entitled, and measures taken to protect your privacy.

4. Medication Error

Years ago, when you saw the doctor, you were closely followed for one or two prescribed medications. Adverse interactions were rare. Today, many people over the age of fifty are taking at least four or five medications; some may take up to fifteen different drugs daily. Over 3.5 billion prescriptions are filled annually in the United States, from among 20,000 prescription drugs.(5) Given the size of these numbers, it is not surprising that medication error is one of the most pressing concerns in health care today. The Institute of Medicine reports that medication errors injure or kill over 1.5 million people annually. These critical mistakes are preventable and involve both prescription drugs and over the counter products, including vitamins, minerals, or herbal supplements. Errors occur in all steps of the medication process, including:

- Prescribing errors at the point of care when health-care professionals send handwritten prescriptions to the pharmacy that are illegible, resulting in misinterpretation of the medication or the dosage when the order is transcribed. Prescribing errors also happen your team of health-care professionals do not communicate with one another.
- Drug-handling errors when full-strength medications are not diluted properly in the pharmacy.
- Drug dispensing errors, where the wrong medication is given to the patient.
- Packaging and labeling errors, when drugs with similar names, abbreviations, or packaging are confused. Look-alike and sound-alike drug names and abbreviations cause products to be mistaken, resulting in the wrong medication or dose given to a patient. Although the FDA has been working with pharmaceutical companies on this problem, it is complicated and not easily resolved.

In a community hospital in Tennessee, Dr. Hills ordered the medication lithium for Jim, an elderly patient who was hospitalized for bipolar disorder. Dr. Hills handwrote the prescription for lithium that went through the hospital system to the pharmacy. The pharmacist had difficulty understanding the doctor's handwriting, read the instructions incorrectly, and sent up a similarly named drug, Librium, which is used for anxiety and not for bipolar disorder.

A patient can safely take 300–600 milligrams of lithium more often and multiple times a day; however, the recommended dose of Librium for elderly people is 5 milligrams two to four times a day. Jim was given 300 milligrams of Librium, 60 times the safe dose. A nurse discovered the mistake a day later, when she noted that Jim was lethargic. Fortunately, he was taken off the medication and survived unharmed.

What You Can Do to Avert Medication Error

- Always keep a list of medications you take. Include the dose, how often you take them, the imprint on each tablet or capsule, and the name of the pharmacy. The imprint can help you identify a drug when you get refills. When your medications change, you must change your list. Enter the changes into your Personal Health Record. Be sure to include over-the-counter medications, vitamins, nutritional supplements, or herbal products you take regularly.

- Keep medications in their original containers. Many pills look alike, so be sure to always be able to distinguish among them.

- Turn on the lights and read the label every time you take a dose to make sure you have the right drug and you are following the instructions.

- Store your medication in a cool dry place out of the reach of children and pets. Be sure that you keep tubes of ointments and creams with medications away from your toothpaste. A mistake could be serious.

- Crush up old medications, mix them with kitty litter or some other substance that will not endanger the environment, and throw them away in the trash. Drugs can become toxic after the expiration date. The shelf life of most drugs is no longer than one year from the date they were filled by the pharmacist.

- Do not chew, crush, or break any capsules or tablets unless there are instructions on the materials that come with the prescriptions directing you to do so. Some long-acting medications are absorbed too quickly when chewed, and other medications won't be effective or could make you sick.

- Use only the cup or measuring device that comes with liquid medication so that you do not chance a dosing error.

- Develop a daily routine for taking your medications and always follow that routine.

- When you get refills of your medications, make sure they look just like the pills you had been taking. If they do not, have a talk with your pharmacist to be sure that you were not erroneously given the wrong medication.

- Make sure all of your doctors know about any allergies and adverse reactions you have had to medicine. Include that information in your PHR.
- When you pick up your medication from the pharmacy, ask the attendant to make sure that it is the drug that your doctor prescribed. Also be sure to take advantage of the opportunity to ask the pharmacist questions about the directions for taking the medication if you are at all uncertain.

Compliance

Caroline is a sixty-year-old woman who loves to cook and spend time with her granddaughter. She suffers from high blood pressure and diabetes. Caroline sees her doctor every three months and fills the prescriptions he gives her at a local pharmacy. However, she readily admits that she does not remember to take her blood pressure medication unless she develops a headache.

Following instructions about taking medication is complex. You go to the doctor and are diagnosed with a simple virus and a cough, and then walk away with three different medications. The instructions about how to take each, when to take each, how to separate taking the different medications, which ones need to be taken with food, etc. are totally confusing so that you could easily take the wrong dosage at the wrong time. It is clear that when you communicate with your physician or physician's assistant and work together to map out a treatment together, you will better understand and follow the directions and have more success in controlling your illness.

The New England Journal of Medicine reported that in 2005, 33–69 percent of medication-related hospital admissions in the United States were due to poor medication adherence with a resultant cost to the American public of over $100 billion a year. The article indicated that among patients with chronic conditions, adherence to a medication regimen drops radically after six months. Among patients taking antidepressants, over half of them stop taking the drugs three months after the initiation of therapy. (6)

You might fail to take prescribed medication correctly because of forgetfulness, confusion about how to take it, unwillingness or inability to assume the cost of the prescription, concerns about potential adverse reactions, previous experience with adverse reaction to medications, lack of information or understanding about how to use a specific remedy, or assuming that because you are feeling better, you no longer need the medication.

Some of the ways to avoid non-adherence are as follows:
- Tell your doctor you want to know the names of your medications and the reasons you are taking them. Make sure that you have full understanding before you leave the physician's office.
- Discuss with your physician the cost of your medication and the financial burden you face to see if there are alternative treatments that you could better afford.
- Request information about your medications or go to the Internet and research the drug.

Electronic Prescribing (E-prescribing)

With nearly four billion prescriptions issued annually in the United States, prescribing medicine is a physician's most frequently used tool for addressing patient problems. The proper distribution of these drugs has a profound effect on the outcome of your treatment. Many physicians write a prescription on a pad of paper and hand it to you. You then go to your local pharmacy to fill the prescription. Many of you use mail-order drug companies for ongoing prescriptions. However, when you are given new medication, there is little time left during the office visit to discuss the impact and side effects of the drugs. As a result, you must learn about your medications from the written informational sheet supplied by the pharmacy or by doing a search on a drug database on the Internet. This process is inefficient and error-prone and not always obvious.

Ellen is a fifty-year-old woman who takes six different medications for mild depression, reflux disease, and chronic asthma. At her annual visit, Ellen and her doctor review her medications. The doctor makes adjustments and, with a new e-prescribing system, sends Ellen's prescriptions directly to a pharmacy located a couple of blocks from her home. Thirty minutes later, Ellen picks

up her medications, packaged with comprehensive instructions. She asks the
pharmacist a couple of questions and leaves feeling completely informed about
what she has to take, when, and how often.

E-prescribing is defined as entering a prescription into an automated
data entry system (handheld, PC, or other) and generating a prescription
electronically. It is based on computer technology that has the capability
to enter, modify, review, and communicate drug prescriptions between the
doctor or nurse practitioner and the pharmacist. In more sophisticated
e-prescribing systems, the computer uses its built-in clinical decision
support to check which medications you are currently taking, whether
or not a new prescription is covered by your health plan, what possible
drug-drug interactions might occur, whether or not the dosage is
appropriate, whether or not you have a history of allergies to anything in
the drug being prescribed, and any other factors that are relevant in the
administration of your medication. When you arrive at the pharmacy to
pick up a prescription, detailed instructions on how to take the medication
are included. E-prescribing speeds the process of dispensing medication
and provides the cross communication among you, your doctor, and your
pharmacist. It results in safer medical practices and helps control costs by
prompting your doctors to select generic drugs that are less expensive.

E-prescribing has proven to be so effective in curbing medication errors
that the Center for Medicare and Medicaid (CMS) has developed a
bonus incentive program that encourages your physicians to implement
e-prescribing and after 2012 will institute a penalty to those physicians
who fail to e-prescribe.

Using Online Pharmacies

*Diane is fifty-seven, and she lives alone in a small home in Burbank, Iowa.
Although she is mobile and able to care for herself, she suffers from diabetes
and hypertension and requires five medications daily to keep her healthy. Her
doctor arranged to have her order and manage her prescriptions through a
state-licensed online service that has a digital copy of her medication profile,
insurance information, and conditions and allergies. An online pharmacist
communicates with Diane by phone and e-mail, and she is able to ask questions*

and access Internet resources that he recommends. All of her pharmaceutical products are mailed to her so she does not have to leave her home.

Online pharmacies provide an invaluable service to patients who are elderly, disabled, or live in remote areas. Those online systems used by insurance companies save you money for three-month orders and are generally as reputable as your local pharmacy. However, some health websites are outright scams. In late 2005, US federal drug investigators shut down 4,600 illegal Internet pharmacy sites and arrested 18 people. Many of these sites purport to offer prescriptions by legitimate doctors following "safe and secure" online diagnoses that typically take the form of a short questionnaire. The scam sites lead the unwary subscriber to believe that their health form is reviewed by a physician before being sent on to a pharmacist, who fills the prescription. In reality, many of the websites fill the orders or send them to an illegal wholesaler without any health-care professional involved.

There are ways for you to save money on prescription medication via online resources. The Veterans Administration enables veterans to refill prescriptions online as a part of the VA's MyHealtheVet service. Five states—Illinois, Kansas, Wisconsin, Vermont, and Missouri—have implemented an online drug program, I-SaveRx, that allows citizens to purchase cheaper, safe prescription drugs from state-approved pharmacies in the United States, Europe, and Canada. With the exception of these few programs, there are hazards to online medication purchases, and before using them, you should check the FDA guidelines regarding the use of online prescription fulfillment services at www.fda.gov/buyonline.

Resources for Safe Health-Care and Medication Advice

www.ahrq.gov/consumer/5steps.htm

www.fda.gov/medwatch/how.htm2.

www.ismp.org/pages/consumer.html

www.medmarx.com

www.nabp.net

Key Points

1. Resources are now available on the web to check the credentials of physicians and the ratings of hospitals. You need to choose a doctor you are comfortable with, who exceeds your expectations when you are ill by being available and answering all of your questions. This is a matter of your medical safety and not just a whimsical desire. If you have to go into the hospital, you want to choose an institution that has an exemplary record for patient safety and a long history of handling the procedures or surgery that you face.

2. Medical errors are all too prevalent. As an e-Patient, you can take responsibility for your health by fully participating and, for example, creating a personal health record that is available to all of your providers and asking questions when you do not understand a treatment or medication.

3. Medication error is the most egregious shortcoming in the medical system, and both patients and providers are responsible. You must always have a list of all your medications available when you are seeking care. You must take it upon yourself to understand the side effects and your allergies to medication. You must be organized about how you store and administer your medication and must adhere to the treatment plan that you have agreed upon with your physicians.

4. You have the right to know what is going on with your health, including results of tests. If you do not understand something, ask your doctor to explain and provide resources for further research, as well as what follow-up is required to resolve your problem.

5. Online pharmacies can serve a valuable purpose, particularly for individuals who are homebound or live in remote areas and are unable to access their medication unless it is sent through the mail. However, as with everything on the web, there are good and bad websites. Patients need to be coached in how to distinguish among them.

Notes

1. Sorrel King, mother of Josie King and founder of the Josie King Foundation, in an interview with the author. For more information on the Josie King Foundation, go to http://www.josieking.org
2. Institute of Medicine, "To Err Is Human: Building a Safer Health System," *Errors in Healthcare: A Leading Cause of Death and Injury,* National Academy Press, 2000, p. 26.
3. Centers for Disease Control and Prevention, National Center for Health Statistics *Deaths: Preliminary Data for 1998, 1999.* National Vital Statistics Reports, Washington D.C. Department of Health and Human Services.
4. Rosemary Gibson, and Singh Janardan Prasad, "A Million Deaths a Decade," *Wall of Silence: The Untold Story of the Medical Mistakes That Kill and Injure Millions of Americans,* Lifeline Press, 2003, p. 41
5. New England Healthcare Institute, "Report on Patient Medication Adherence," Med Ad News, February 2010. http://www.nehi.net.
6. Lars OsterbergMD, and Terrence Blaschke, MD, "Adherence to Medication," New England Journal of Medicine, 353(2005):487–497.

Chapter Six

Receiving Care across Geographic Boundaries

Never before in history has innovation offered promise of so much to so many in so short a time.

Bill Gates, <u>Business @ the Speed of Thought: Using a Digital Nervous System</u> with Collins Hemingway Warner Books, 1999.

On November 21, 2004, eighteen-month-old baby Kate was critically injured in a car accident. She was rushed by paramedics to the closest hospital in Douglas, Arizona, a small rural town along the US-Mexico border. Kate was in shock and minutes away from death, having lost almost two-thirds of her blood from multiple injuries. The nearest trauma center was in Tucson, more than a hundred miles away. When she arrived at the Douglas emergency room, the doctor saw immediately that he would need assistance and called the University Medical Center's Level 1 Trauma Center in Tucson. Over the Arizona Telemedicine Program (ATP) network, a trauma surgeon at UMC was able to see the baby and examine her injuries. He reviewed the Kate's vital signs, X-rays, and lab tests results and virtually led the doctors and nurses in Douglas through emergency medical procedures. Once Kate was resuscitated and stabilized, she was transported to the UMC for further treatment. She fully recovered (1)

Patients are scattered throughout areas of the country far removed from major medical institutions. It is estimated by the American Medical Association that there are more than thirty-five million Americans who live in medically underserved areas, and it would take sixteen thousand additional doctors nationwide to provide services to them. If these individuals are injured in an accident or become critically ill, they stand a far greater chance of facing death than a person with similar conditions in an urban area where there is easy access to a major medical center. With physician and nurse shortages, fewer medical school graduates selecting primary care medicine, and a rapidly growing senior population that requires more and more medical services as they age, telemedicine offers a better way to provide access to comprehensive health services that are needed.

Baby Adam is born at the Hays Medical Center in Kansas with a suspected heart murmur. There is no pediatric cardiologist on staff there; however, at Hays, patients' radiology films are automatically transferred to specialists in Wichita, Kansas, where they are read instantly, and a diagnosis is sent back in hours not days. Within moments of birth, using an electronic stethoscope, Adam's heartbeat is transmitted to the pediatric cardiologist, who is 270 miles away. With a video hookup, he is able to help the Hays cardiology technician do an echocardiogram, which provides the data to make a diagnosis, advise the local doctors on the best possible care for Adam, and reassure the boy's parents that the problem is being appropriately handled. (2)

The convergence of the Internet, high-bandwidth telecommunications, video technology, sophisticated medical robots, and the spread of electronic health records provide the enabling technologies for computer-based diagnostics that connect you with your doctors or connect a local primary care physician with a specialist who could be separated geographically by hundreds or thousands of miles. This technology enables you to receive high quality care without travelling great distances in the event of a catastrophic illness or emergency. It enables you to connect with super-specialists using interactive audio and video conferencing, as well as high-speed telephone lines that can send lab tests, X-rays, and vital signs, then almost instantly receive a diagnosis and treatment plan. There is video technology that enables face-to-face examination and allows you to receive physical therapy, occupational and mental health treatment, and hospice services remotely. There are services available to homebound individuals to monitor chronic conditions hourly or daily.

In many remote areas in Arizona, the Dakotas, Idaho, Montana, Oregon, Washington, and Wyoming, telemedicine technology now enables patients to access needed medical services. Dozens of asthmatic children in these areas use web cams in their homes to send videos showing how they use their inhalers and send readings from their peak flow meters (airflow measurement devices) to pulmonary specialists located at major medical centers. Diabetic patients on Indian reservations in rural Arizona now have their retinas screened and treated remotely by ophthalmologists at world-renowned eye centers throughout the country for diabetic eye changes that could lead to complications and blindness. Telemedicine also has other benefits, such as enabling emergency care and keeping family members in the loop when patients are transported to distant hospitals.

Twin babies born in rural Washington State went into distress shortly after their birth and were transported immediately by helicopter to the closest large neonatal care center 140 miles away. Their mother had not even been able to see her babies before they were flown out. Since she had three other children at home, it was virtually impossible for her to go with her newborn twins. Northwest Telehealth, a telemedicine network of Inland Northwest Health Services in Spokane, Washington, arranged for a telephone connection with video screens between the mother and her babies. For six weeks, using a telehealth camera, the mom could see her one-pound babies, watch them receive a feeding, hear them burp, and enjoy their first smiles while tending to the immediate needs of the others in her family. This bonding could never be replaced after the fact.

Teletherapy

Bob is a farmer who lives in rural Minnesota. He was severely burned on his hands, chest, and back while fixing some farm machinery. He was treated initially in a local hospital and, after he was stable, transferred to the Regional Burn Center in Rochester, Minnesota, 450 miles from his home. Once he was released, Bob arranged for his follow-up care to be handled over the St. Alexius Telecare network of North Dakota. He participated in three telemedicine visits, each lasting thirty minutes, avoiding a two-day trip that would have necessitated leaving the farm with no one in charge during harvest time. This long-distance care enabled Bob to keep the farm going. It also provided relief to the family, because they did not have to transport him 450 miles and back. (4)

Speech Therapy

It was a typical spring day on May 27 for Wes, who worked at a National Guard camp in North Dakota. Suddenly he collapsed while using a mini front loader. He was taken to the local Carrington Health Center, where he was diagnosed with a ruptured brain aneurysm. He was immediately flown to Fargo, North Dakota, where doctors were able to keep Wes alive without surgery. After seventeen days in the hospital and another twenty-seven days in rehab, Wes was able to return home. Doctors recommended that he continue with physical therapy, occupational therapy, and speech therapy; however, speech therapy was not available at Carrington Health Center near his home. With a telemedicine connection from St. Alexius Medical Center, Wes was able to have the therapy, which made him physically more comfortable and capable, and mentally and emotionally more confident. Wes returned to work full time one year after his collapse. Without the therapy, he would not have been able to continue work at all. (5)

St. Alexius is one example of a full service hospital with seventeen affiliated clinics located in remote areas of North and South Dakota. The St. Alexius telemedicine network has been functioning for ten years, and it enables doctors to see patients who would otherwise not be served by specialists, and in some cases, not even by primary care physicians. Using the network, St. Alexius doctors conduct between four hundred and five hundred consults every year, including twenty-four-seven trauma consultations between the emergency room at St. Alexius and outlying centers. Much of the work they do includes post-operative and post-trauma care, similar to what Bob received. For example, doctors at St. Alexius are able to remotely check a patient's incision while the patient remains in the home. St. Alexius also offers speech therapy to stroke patients, diabetes and Alzheimer support groups, and mental health services that would be unavailable otherwise. Sometimes they even use the equipment to resolve a personal crisis. (3)

There are many other centers of excellence offering telemedicine care. Marshfield Clinic in Marshfield, Wisconsin, has over 775 physicians in more than 80 medical specialties and subspecialties located in 54 locations throughout northern, central, and western Wisconsin. An integral part of health care delivery at Marshfield Clinic is the Outreach Services program. More than 1,200 hospitals, clinics, and other sites participate in these outreach programs. Clinic physicians and staff provide off-site consultation in 52 specialties. The clinic had more than 3.8 million patient encounters for the year ended September 30, 2010, and reported 376,708 unique patients in the clinic system during this same period.

Examples of its services include off-site physician consultation involving more than 80 sub—specialties, twenty-four-hour EKG interpretation via computer, mobile echocardiography, a reference laboratory, regional blood banking, radiology, EEGs, orthotics and prosthetics, radiation physics, pulmonary function, and biomedical electronics.

A telehealth visit at Marshfield Clinic is scheduled by telephone. A specific provider for a patient is selected based on the patient's individual problem. At the appointed time, a trained telehealth nurse-clinician orients the patient, who is at a local clinic, to the telehealth consult process and prepares the patient and family for a clinical exam. The provider and patient can see and hear each other, just as if they were sitting in the same room. The doctor is on TV, and the patient and family are in an exam room with the nurse practitioner, perhaps a hundred miles away. During the exam, specially designed equipment gives the doctor all the information needed to make a diagnosis and to discuss a plan of care with the patient and the family. Handheld cameras can zoom in for tight close-ups to give the doctor a good picture. Digital stethoscopes with headphones that intensify sounds of the heart and lungs enable the doctor to listen to the heart; fiber optic cameras allow doctors to "see" inside the ears, eyes, and mouth. Doctors use a clinical-quality video system on the computer to conduct the consultation. The precision of these instruments allows the doctor to make a diagnosis as if doctor and patient were in the same room. Everyone can talk back and forth during these exams, and questions are encouraged. (4)

Physical Therapy

Physical therapy services delivered remotely are also convenient and efficient for providing services to disabled patients who live in rural locations or are housebound. With available digital technology, there is no need for the patient and health care professional to be in the same location. Internet-based videoconferencing installed right at the patient's bedside in the home or in a local physician's clinic will enable a physical and occupational therapists to assess the physical condition of a patient, communicate remedial movements or remedial sustained postures, and evaluate the patient's progress over time. The therapist is also able to instruct patients to move in a particular manner, to assume a sustained posture, or perform a test. The patient and the distant health-care provider are able to see each other in full color and hear each other using full-motion video and digital audio systems. This technology has proven successful for acute stroke care and for rehabilitation following surgery or severe injury.

A twenty-five-year-old woman suffered a brain injury and was in a rehabilitation center. Her insurance ran out, and she was discharged to her home in a remote section of Oklahoma. The family was unable to care for her without help and training. They were introduced to a teletherapy program through INTEGRIS Health in Oklahoma City that provides access to medical care for rural Oklahomans and others. A physical therapist worked with family members using phone connections and cameras to teach the patient how to move about. At the beginning of the teletherapy, the patient could not sit in a wheelchair without assistance. At the end of twelve weeks, she was walking around the home with little assistance and able to do a number of life skills for herself.(5)

Mental Health Services

According to the National Institute of Mental Health, an estimated 26.2 percent of Americans age eighteen and older, about one in four adults, suffer from a mental disorder in a given year. In addition, NIMH reports that mental disorders are the leading cause of disability in the United States and Canada for ages fifteen to forty-four. Many people suffer from more than one mental disorder at a given time. Nearly half (45 percent) of those with any mental disorder meet criteria for two or more disorders. (6)

There is a severe lack of mental health services throughout the United States, and the problem is especially acute in rural areas. Telemedicine—appointments by video screen and telephone—are increasingly used by psychiatrists to provide counseling to many who would otherwise be unable to get help. A simple audio telephone connection or video system is all that is needed for a specialist to consult with patients who lives miles away.

A woman from Arkansas, left destitute with four children to support, was clinically depressed and in danger of losing her children. A local nurse contacted a physician connected to the Rural Arkansas Delta Integrated Telehealth system in Little Rock, Arkansas. He arranged for a consultation with a University of Arkansas psychologist. Since she had limited income and no phone or transportation, the local police transported her to a facility near her home where she was able to receive her telehealth consultations with a psychologist over interactive video equipment. With this counseling, the woman was able to function and take care of her children.

Traumas and Emergencies

In trauma medicine, split-second timing can mean the difference between life and death, between the ability to save or lose a limb, between a short-term injury and long-term recurrent problems. With telemedicine providing fast access to trauma specialists, countless people have been saved from prolonged pain, suffering, and even death as they await a diagnosis or a transfer. By enabling trained emergency technicians and nurses to act immediately to control bleeding, administer appropriate medications, suture wounds, and care for patients with assistance from the specialists looking on through the eye of the camera and making the diagnosis or providing instructions, lives are being saved.

Martin, who worked at a lumber mill in northern California, caught his hand and forearm in the chain that moved wood through the mill. A local family nurse practitioner assessed the injury and sent images to the Santa Rosa Memorial Hospital Emergency Department for a telemedicine assessment and consult with the emergency physician and a radiologist. Based on the consult, the nurse practitioner was able to clean, suture, and splint the wound, and Martin avoided a five-hour round trip to the hospital and unnecessary transport costs. (7)

In a unique program forged between fourteen community hospitals and the Massachusetts General Hospital Telestroke service, trained neurologists now treat stroke patients via a telemedicine network that brings the specialists to the bedside of the patient during those critical first three hours. These specialists work with local physicians to help them diagnose whether the symptoms they are seeing are indeed stroke and the best way to address the problem. Many similar telestroke centers are emerging throughout the nation.

Telehospice: Death with Dignity

Hospice administers a range of health and comfort care services to patients who are nearing the end of life. A much misunderstood and underused service, hospice enables terminal patients to die as they wish at home. Hospice attempts to meet the needs of this population with services such as pain management, spiritual counseling, helping people to get paperwork in order, and providing reassurance to the family. The availability of telemonitoring workstation equipment that is already being used to monitor many homebound patients enables patients to transition to telehospice care. There is much technology available today, including telecommunications-ready infusion pumps for pain management and videotapes for caregiver education, that at the touch of a button can make a huge difference.

Online Second Opinion Consults

A fifty-five-year-old man living in a small town in New Mexico was diagnosed with a growth lodged in his abdomen. There was no indication of whether or not this growth was benign or a cancer. Primary care doctors and specialists all had different opinions as to what to do. One suggested a biopsy, another suggested surgery, and a third wanted to wait. With all of the confusion, the man decided to seek a second opinion and opted to contact the Mayo Clinic for advice. Flying to the Mayo Clinic, located in Rochester, Wisconsin, meant time away from work and an expensive trip, so the patient opted for a second opinion online via telemedicine. The existence of an electronic medical record, video and audio high-speed transmission, and the ability to send films and lab reports ahead to the specialists at the Mayo Clinic combined to make this consultation possible and successful.

With certain diagnoses, such as heart disease, cancer, autoimmune disorders, and other serious illnesses, you often get mixed messages and several different opinions. Using telemedicine technology, you can get a second opinion from leading specialists in hours without having to wait agonizing months and travel great distances for an appointment. Many companies have incorporated online second opinion consultations into their employee benefit packages that you might be able to take advantage of. There are channels available when illness strikes that enable you to access the best specialists throughout the country to resolve mixed messages and differing diagnoses and help you through the confusion of what to do.

Legal Issues

One of the impediments to the practice of telemedicine has been state licensure regulations that prohibit doctors from practicing medicine across state lines. Physicians who wish to participate in telemedicine consults must receive authorization by their State Boards of Registration in Medicine in order to engage in these activities beyond the boundaries of that practice's state lines. Federal legislation passed in 2007 now mandates that if you live in a remote an area that is defined as a health practice shortage area (HPSA), where there are severe shortages of primary care physicians, dentists, and mental health practitioners, you can access the services of remote doctors, nurses, nurse practitioners, physician's assistants, clinical nurse specialists, nurse anesthetists, nurse midwives, social workers, or clinical psychologists, who will be reimbursed for their efforts. The legislation includes only interactive telemedicine encounters. The reimbursement is 75 percent of the rate of an in-person consultation.

Poor reimbursement can also be a deterrent among physicians and slow down the spread of telemedicine to places where it is needed. Payment policies vary from state to state and are slowly evolving. The Center for Medicare and Medicaid Services (CMS) now allows reimbursement for telemedicine interactions at the discretion of individual state health-care agencies when they prove to be a more cost-effective alternative than the traditional face-to-face consultation or examination.

Home Telemonitoring

One out of every eight persons is over the age of sixty-five in the United States. By the year 2030, that number will double, accounting for 25 percent of the population. These baby boomers face the double challenge of caring for elderly parents while dealing with their own emerging health problems as they approach retirement. With the shortage of doctors and nurses in America, millions of individuals will be able to help their elderly parents, themselves, and their children with the assistance of telemonitoring. Telemonitoring services enable you to check your blood pressure, heart rate, weight, and blood glucose, and then send objective data to clinicians over the telephone or through an Internet connection from your home. The wireless systems used in home monitoring are predicated upon a set of noninvasive, wearable monitors (many available for reimbursement), such as the following:

- A blood pressure cuff with a telecommunications plug-in and a similar device to monitor blood glucose are attached to a telehealth computer workstation. The telehealth work station is connected to your phone line and is linked through the line to a computer at a hospital or clinic, where a nurse monitors the readings.
- A desktop glass ball called an orb can be set to glow different colors based on preprogrammed instructions when used in conjunction with a smart pillbox. This helps you adhere to a schedule of taking medications by sending a signal from the pillbox to the orb, which glows red when a medication is overdue and green when you are

on schedule with your medications. The smart pillbox sends an electronic message to a central server that houses your data. The server then signals back to the orb.

- An implantable cardioverter defibrillator (ICD) notifies your doctor each time it gives you a jolt to stop a potentially dangerous abnormal heart rhythm.

- A recorder the size of a computer mouse gathers data from your pacemaker or ICD. When you hold it to your chest, the device sends the number to a secure computer that you or your doctor can access via the Internet.

- A watch checks your blood sugar levels through the skin and transmits the readings to a remote site, where a nurse or nurse's assistant is monitoring the input.

- A soft machine-washable undershirt can take a continuous movie of your heart's electrical activity, blood pressure, oxygen level, and other health indicators.

- A ring the size of a college class ring continuously measures body temperature, heart rate, and oxygen levels in the blood and sends this information to a cell phone or computer.

- A wireless electronic bathroom scale sends weight data into a home monitoring system (a device the size of a phone answering machine) programmed to flash if the patient forgets to check in.

- A similarly constructed wireless blood pressure cuff sends blood pressure readings to the device, which then sends these readings directly to a computer at a doctor's office or clinic, where a nurse or case manager will review it.

To keep in touch with his nurses, eighty-year-old Ed has been using a home monitoring system with two-way video for many years. Each morning, he steps on a mat that records his weight. A bracelet sensor reads his blood pressure, heart rate, and oxygen levels. These indicators are sent via a telephone connection to a group of nurses at a remote location, and if there is an irregularity, they video teleconference with Ed. Using an electronic stethoscope, they can listen to his heart and talk with him about what might be wrong. If the problem looks serious, Ed is advised to go to the hospital. The home monitoring crew alerts the hospital staff that he is coming and provides them with the details of his condition. Most times, hospital visits are not necessary, and all that is needed is a simple adjustment of Ed's medications.

With remote phone or video consultations such as those that Ed uses, every patient who is located in a rural area where medical services are not easily available, as well as patients who live in urban areas but are homebound, can self manage many of their health issues. The technology also enables your providers to remotely identify the onset of complications and give you an action remedy right away or determine that you must travel the distance to come in to see them. When you do get to a physician's office or the emergency department, your consistent home monitoring provides the baseline information for a quick assessment of what is wrong. All of this eliminates many of those costly, frightening emergency room visits.

Hays Telemedicine in Hays, Kansas, conducted a study on congestive heart failure in patients who were monitored at home by telemedicine nurses. These patients were seen weekly using a modified television in the home connected to a television cable system base station. At the base station, a telemedicine nurse monitored the study participants. Home and office visits were prescheduled, and when a home intervention was required to draw blood or do other lab tests, someone from the Visiting Nurses Association made the home visit and collected the necessary data. The study showed that the patients had 20 percent fewer emergency room visits; they were more likely to remain in their homes instead of going to a nursing home; and there was a significant cost savings to the individuals and to the system. (8)

Implementing a Home Monitoring System

There are several criteria for you to be considered for a home monitoring system that is reimbursed by health insurance, Medicare, or Medicaid:
- You must have a disability.
- You must have impaired ability to care for yourself.
- You must be recovering from an illness, surgery, or hospital stay.
- You must be living with a chronic illness that is poorly controlled.
- You must have a terminal illness.

Additional home services range from skilled medical care to home support services, or a combination of both. Skilled care is directed by your doctor and is provided by health care professionals such as nurses, medical social workers, and physical therapists. It can include activities such as home dialysis, drawing blood, administering medication, and physical and occupational therapy. Home support services help you with basic everyday issues such as dressing and bathing, and are provided by home health aides.

Finding Home Care Services That Are Right for You

The first step to finding a home care service is to talk to your doctor or other health-care professionals, such as physical or occupational therapists or social workers. If you are looking for a reputable home health care agency, a hospital social worker or nurse may be able to help. Other sources include your state and county health department, local agencies on aging, and the national Eldercare Locator, a public service of the Administration on Aging. Once you find a home health-care service that you think will satisfy your needs, questions to ask about their qualifications to assist in making a decision include:

- How long has the agency been in business?
- Is the agency approved by your health maintenance organization or supplemental insurance?
- Is the agency evaluated and accredited by a governing body such as the Joint Commission's Home Care Accreditation Program or Medicare?
- Is the agency licensed by the state? (Most states require agencies to be licensed and reviewed regularly, and the report is available upon request through the health department.)
- Can the agency provide references (a list of doctors, hospitals, discharge planners, and former clients)?
- What are the credentials of the providers who work with this agency?
- Does the agency make clear its policies regarding billing, services, and fees?
- Does the agency provide any resources that will help you with financial assistance for their services?
- Are there days of exclusion before your coverage will begin?
- How many hours of coverage each week are allocated, and is there twenty-four-hour coverage for emergencies?

- Does the agency involve you or your family in planning your care and making adjustments? Do they require involvement of a family member and specify what is required of that individual?
- Is there a program for conflict resolution and a clearly defined process for answering your questions or complaints?
- Do they provide and service special equipment such as oxygen, respirators, dialysis, and train you in how to use the equipment?

Among the ways that home health-care services get paid for are:

Medicare: Medicare may pay for medical home health-care services through a certified home health-care agency if a physician orders these services. Services covered by Medicare include skilled nursing assistance or physical, speech, or occupational therapy. If your home health services are covered under Medicare, your doctor, care manager, or discharge planner will probably make arrangements for a home health-care agency.

Medicaid: Depending on your income and assets, anyone is eligible.

Older Americans Act: This federal program funds state and local programs that provide services to frail and disabled individuals who are sixty years old or older.

Veterans Affairs: If you are a veteran and at least 50 percent disabled due to a service-related injury or illness, you may be eligible for medical services through Veterans Affairs hospital-based home care services.

Community Organizations: Depending on your situation and finances, certain community organizations cover home care costs.

Insurance: Many insurance programs cover some home health-care services for short-term medical needs. However, long-term coverage varies. Long-term care policies are available through private insurance companies and the federal government.

The eICU®: Remote Monitoring for Intensive Care

If you are unlucky enough to land in the intensive care unit, you have cause for concern. With a severe shortage of ICU specialists, the expertise that an intensive care doctor brings to the critical care unit is missing in many hospitals. Fewer than six thousand intensivists are actively practicing in the United States, leaving only 13 percent of ICU patients receiving dedicated intensivist care. With the aging population and its anticipated need for intensive care, the acute shortage of specialists compounds the problem. When an intensive care doctor is available to manage the ICU, studies show that a patient's chance of dying in the ICU decreases by 30 percent.

The eICU® is a central command room outfitted with cameras that beam directly to each patient's bedside. Broadband technologies and land-based wireless networks allow continuous communication of data, voice, and video at ultra high speeds. The eICU® can be located within a hospital complex or offsite at a completely different location minutes or miles from the intensive care unit. It is manned twenty-four-seven by intensive care doctors and nurses. All of the information that the doctor needs to make a decision comes directly into the eICU®. From a control station, several computer screens display your diagnosis and progress, doctors' notes, and vital signs such as heart rate and blood pressure. The equipment enables the eICU® doctor to see your medical record, including nurse's notes and blood test results. Video conferencing equipment enables two-way conversation between the eICU doctor and you and your family. The eICU® doctor is also able to zoom in on you and gauge your level of consciousness. This helps the doctor by providing much more information than an average doctor or specialist on call would have. Dedicated hot phones create an instantaneous link between each ICU in the network and the care team in the eICU®. The constant surveillance arms the ICU physician with the patient information needed to make the right decisions. Many large and small hospitals throughout the nation now use the eICU® as a safer, more efficient way to monitor their patients.

Telemedicine and Health-Care Costs

One of your biggest health-care concerns is the cost of your health care and how to keep it under control. Telemedicine promises to play a key role in solving some of the cost issues inherent in the face-to-face delivery of medical care that has been the norm. One of the major benefits of telemedicine is to reduce the number of patient visits to doctor's offices, clinics, and hospitals. Those visits could involve the transfer of individuals from nursing homes, correctional facilities, and local hospitals to trauma centers. Not only are these transfers expensive, but sometimes they are wasted effort. Many of the issues that require transport are easily handled by home monitoring and telephone consultations. Monitoring the vital signs of individuals with chronic disease such as congestive heart failure and diabetes has the potential to reduce the country's health-care costs by several billion dollars over the next twenty-five years. Those savings would come from spotting problems before they develop, thus reducing emergency department visits, preventing hospitalizations, and cutting the length of hospital stays.

Research from the Center for Information Technology Leadership (CITL) confirms that the practice of telemedicine saves money. Their study, *The Value of Provider-to-Provider Telehealth Technologies*, examines the cost-benefit of using telemedicine/telehealth technologies, such as real-time video and store-and-forward data capture in emergency rooms, correctional institutions, nursing homes, and physician offices. It concludes that if a telemedicine initiative were nationally implemented for a period of five years, the savings could be $4.28 billion per year. The study goes on to state that because it only considered telemedicine in certain settings and not others, its findings may be conservative. (9)

Telemedicine for the Greater Good

It is clear that widespread deployment of telemedicine has many potential benefits, like greater access to doctors for individuals who live in areas where medical clinicians are not always available, a large reduction in the numbers of people who are forced to live in institutional settings because there is no other way for them to obtain needed health services, and immediate emergency medicine expertise in trauma cases that occur far away from hospitals and emergency departments. Telemedicine also promises to greatly reduce care costs for millions of individuals and for the health-care system using continuous monitoring that keeps people stable and averts a crisis. Just as e-Patients have aggressively pursued their quest for health-care information online to address their individual illnesses and conditions, e-Patients must investigate and actively pursue telemedicine applications and home monitoring services when and where they are needed.

Key Points

1. Digital technology is now available to provide expert clinician care to patients when distance separates them.
2. Telemedicine depends upon a robust infrastructure that includes the Internet, video, high-speed high-bandwidth telecommunications, computer-based diagnostics, and various medical devices that enable doctors to virtually examine, treat, and interact with patients.
3. Home monitoring is critical to the care of those individuals who have chronic disease or a disability.
4. There are a variety of medical devices that can send vital statistics and other information to your doctors or nurses, who continuously monitor you and can adjust your medications or offer advice from a remote location. This ability will save you from unnecessary visits to your clinician or to emergency rooms.
5. Telemedicine can offer you access to consults and second opinions with key experts from any major medical facility.
6. Telerehabilitation provides you with virtual physical therapy, hearing and speech therapy, occupational therapy, mental health services, and hospice services right in your home.
7. Ongoing maintenance programs such as the monitoring of asthmatic children, providing remote eye exams, and administering telerehabilitation and mental health services reduce the need for emergency medical procedures and save time, money, and the anxiety of having to transport individuals to a care facility.
8. In an emergency, telemedicine can mean the difference between life and death.

9. E-Patients, when considering a hospital admission, might want to find out if the hospital they choose has an intensive care physician on staff or an eICU® program. The eICU® makes it possible for every intensive care unit in a hospital to have a physician who specializes in intensive care medicine checking patients at all times.
10. Private medical institutions, the states, and the federal government have to work together to vastly expand the telemedicine infrastructure so that is more ubiquitous and available.

Notes

1. Arizona Telemedicine Program, "A Life Saved through Teletrauma Service." *Arizona Telemedicine Newsletter* p.4 at:www.federaltelemedicine.com.
2. Robert Cox, MD, Medical Director at Hays Medical Center in Hays, Kansas, in an interview with the author, September 2009.
3. Lisa Vetter, Telemedicine Specialist, St. Alexius Medical Center and Telecare Network of North Dakota, in an interview with the author, October 2009.
4. Nina Antoniotti, Marshfield Clinic, Telehealth Network, Marshfield, Wisconsin, in an interview with the author, February 2010.
5. Edward D. Lemaire, Yvon Boudrias, Gayle Greene, "Low-Bandwidth Internet-Based Videoconferencing for Physical Rehabilitation Consultations," *Telemedicine, Telecare,* Royal Society of Medicine Press, 7(2001):82-89, doi:10.1258/1357633011936200.
6. Statistics from National Institute of Mental Health http://www.apps.nimh.nih.gov/healthstatistics/index.shtml/
7. Health Resources and Services Administration, anecdote from case studies on telehealth, *Consultations Using Telemedicine*, p. 5 http://www.teleHealth.hrsa.gov/grants/success.html.
8. Dr. Robert Cox Medical Director at Hays Medical Center, Hays, Kansas, in an interview with the author.
9. E. Pan, C. Cusack, J. Hook, A. Vincent, D.C. Kaelber, D.W. Bates, and B. Middleton, "The Value of Provider-to-Provider Telehealth Technologies" *Telemedicine Journal E Health* 14, 5(2008):446–53.

Chapter Seven

Patient-Centered Care

In spite of their growing independence, patients still expect to have a close, trusting, and personal relationship with their primary care physicians. They also want to be partners with their doctors.

Lawrence, David, MD, Chairman Emeritus, Kaiser Permanente. From Chaos to Care, Ad Capo Press, 2002, p.14.

A new model of care is evolving—patient-centered care—that creates a health-care team consisting of you, your physician, possibly a physician's assistant or nurse practitioner, your family, and other health-care professionals such as social workers and therapists. This team works together with you to insure that you are receiving the coordinated care appropriate for your particular situation. In past generations, your care was based on your physician's evaluation of your health issues and the treatment recommended. This sea change in the care model now places the responsibility for your health care directly with you, in partnership with your providers. The IOM defines patient-centered care as "providing care that is respectful of and responsive to individual patient preferences, needs, and values and ensuring that patient values guide all clinical decisions." Further the IOM states that "twenty-first century medicine should be care based on continuous health relationships. Patients should receive care whenever they need it and in many forms, not just face-to-face visits." Patient-centered care presupposes several things:

- That you and your family are encouraged to participate in your care.
- That you share in decision making leading to specific actions and treatment.
- That you direct your care, with the advice of your providers, when you are healthy and have a family advocate or friend do so when you are too sick.
- That you get all of the care that you need, within the boundaries of what your health insurance allows.
- That you have choices in determining who your providers will be based on performance data that is available to you.
- That you determine how your health-care dollars are spent by becoming a better health-care shopper who is able to find and evaluate purchases and understand the consequences of your choices.
- That your health-care professionals communicate with you and your family and share complete and unbiased information.
- That the information you receive is timely, complete, and accurate and presented in a way that will help you effectively participate in care decisions.
- That all forms of communication—e-mail, online technologies such as patient portals and discussion forums, clinical information systems, smartphones, and telemonitoring systems—are used in your interactions with your providers.
- That you are granted full access to care, not just via face-to-face and phone consultation, but via e-mail and e-visits during off-hours.
- That there is good communication among physicians, nurses, and other health professionals taking care of you so that medical errors are reduced and duplication of tests and procedures are avoided.(1)

The patient-centered care model requires a major commitment from providers and patients. It considers your cultural traditions, personal preferences, and values; your family situation; and lifestyles. It places responsibility for important aspects of self-care, such as blood-sugar or blood-pressure monitoring, in your hands. It includes the tools and support needed to fulfill those tasks. Multiple studies indicate that you are more likely to take your pills, eliminate bad food from your diet, and show up for appointments when you are encouraged to make your own choices.

Patient-centered care is based upon the premise that there is a provider for every patient—a gatekeeper who coordinates and ensures continuity of care, even under the most extreme circumstances.

Your Medical Team

As we enter the second decade of the twenty-first century, there are nearly fifty thousand fewer primary care doctors in practice than are needed to support the demand for basic medical care in the United States, particularly with legislation that mandates that every American citizen must have health-care coverage. This means that nearly 20 percent of Americans (fifty-six million people) have inadequate or no access to primary care. Unfortunately, medical school graduates continue to choose specialty practice over primary care because the pay is better, the workday is shorter, and the liabilities are fewer. It is your primary care provider, however, who is charged with making sure that your basic care needs are covered, including annual physical exams, vaccinations, appropriate labs, and tests. Your primary care provider is also trained to inform you about good health practices, disease prevention, health maintenance, and treatment of your chronic and acute illnesses. They advise and educate you and coordinate care with all of your specialists, nurses, social workers, and therapists. They provide you with referrals and prescription refills and help you seek a second opinion when appropriate. This is basic health care, and it should be based on a trusted relationship. With the extreme shortage of primary care physicians and little hope that this problem will be resolved in the near future, many health institutions, HMOs, and family and internal medicine practices have turned to physician assistants, or nurse practitioners to help fill the gap.

A physician assistant is a health-care professional licensed to practice medicine with the supervision of a licensed physician. The main focus of a physician assistant is prevention, maintenance of treatment for chronic conditions, education, and collaboration with patients to maximize care efficiency. Physician assistants conduct exams, diagnose and treat illnesses, order and interpret tests, counsel on preventive care, assist in surgery, and write prescriptions. Their education encompasses many of the same science courses and laboratory instruction taught in medical school. The training requires two to three years beyond undergraduate education. A physician assistant must also pass a National Certifying Exam (PANCE) before receiving a license to practice. They are required to earn and log continuing education credits and renew their license every two years. Every six years, they must take an exam for recertification.

Some primary care practices use nurse practitioners to provide basic care services. There are also independently practicing nurse practitioners. These individuals also must have a license to practice, which qualifies them to see patients, give exams, make diagnoses, collaborate with physicians, make referrals, and diagnose and treat acute illness, injuries, and infections. They also write prescriptions, counsel patients on health behaviors, manage chronic conditions, and make referrals to various therapists. Most nurse practitioners specialize in a specific area of medicine (e.g., family medicine, pediatrics, obstetrics and gynecology, or diabetes). Using physician assistants and nurse practitioners is a cost-effective way to maintain effective individualized care, and you can rest assured that they are well qualified to handle your basic medical care and will have time to thoroughly address your concerns. These professionals use the tools of technology, including digital health records, e-mail, smartphones, patient portals, e-visits, and telemedicine, and they communicate with your primary care doctors and specialists. What is important is that you have a central place where you are receiving your basic medical care.

The Patient-Centered Medical Home

With available technology, a new model of care has evolved: the patient-centered medical home (PCMH), where you choose a primary care provider who could be a physician, physician's assistant, or nurse practitioner. Access to a specialist is available when needed. In the PCMH, you are at the center of the health-care experience, supported by your team of caregivers and by the technology. This includes a secure portal, e-mail, and an electronic health record that contains your lab tests and your medical history. Your provider team helps you find links to websites that explain various conditions and enable you to engage in online discussions. You also have the convenience of flexible scheduling, which includes e-visits and e-prescribing. Patients who have a medical home stay healthier. This is because the staff at your medical home is familiar with your medical history and can help with preventative care and managing chronic conditions such as high blood pressure, diabetes, and asthma. Reimbursement in a PCMH model includes not only the usual fee for service payment but a retainer fee system, typically paid by your health insurer, that pays for services associated with coordination of care between your medical home practice, consultants, therapists, and community resources.

The Patient-Centered Primary Care Collaborative is a coalition of employers, consumer groups, health plans, and health-care professionals that promotes the concept of the PCMH. The collaborative conducted several pilot projects with results indicating that patients who had a PCMH had far fewer emergency room visits and hospitalizations. Additionally, among patients with chronic conditions, there was as much as a 40 percent decrease in hospitalizations and nearly 30 percent reduction in ER visits. These patients who had a medical home appeared to stay healthier and experienced significant health-care cost savings. (2)

In 2007, Group Health of Seattle decided to experiment with a PCMH model of care. Group Health reported the following: During the two years studied, the team's patients had 29 percent fewer ER visits and 6 percent fewer hospitalizations compared with other Group Health clinic patients. There were start-up costs—sixteen dollars per patient per year—and it took a couple of years to provide the bulk of the savings. However, for every dollar invested in the system, Group Health saved $1.50 by keeping patients out of the ER and the hospital. Medical home patients reported better care experiences.

The strategy is now being expanded to all twenty-six of Group Health's Washington-state medical centers, covering more than four hundred thousand patients. Home monitoring tools such as weight and blood pressure measurement devices that transmit readings via the Internet both to children of elderly home-bound parents and to a health-care provider enable not only the relatively healthy patient to be a part of the medical home but also provide a way for the elderly to remain in their own homes rather than go to assisted living and nursing home facilities, yet they still have the assurance of being cared for and safe.

The American Academy of Pediatrics (AAP) in a policy statement advocates that every child deserves a medical home where care is accessible, continuous, comprehensive, patient—and family-centered, coordinated, compassionate, and culturally effective. The AAP suggests the following characteristics for a medical home for children:

- Family-centered care based upon a collaborative working partnership with families, respecting their diversity and recognizing that they are the constant in a child's life.
- A community-based system with a coordinated network of services that promote the healthy development of children and includes ongoing primary care as well as access to a broad range of specialty and ancillary services.
- Optimization of the lifelong health that continues uninterrupted as the individual moves through the system from adolescent to adulthood. (3)

Pilot PCMH programs conducted by Medicaid demonstrate that coordinated patient-centered care using the medical home concept contributes real value to care and reduces cost. A Medicaid study documented a savings of $3.5 million over three years for asthma management and $2.1 million savings for a diabetes care initiative. These savings accrued from elimination of wasteful duplication of services, tests, and procedures and from close control of chronic illnesses.(4)

While the medical home is not a silver bullet that will solve all the problems of twenty-first century health care, it has the potential to transform health care by blending personalized care with team-based coordinated care that deploys technology to help you understand and work through complex health-care issues. You have to seek your own medical home, either with the right primary care practice or through a clinic or health center. You also have to do the work to insure that you supply all of the necessary elements for the best patient-centered care available. To do that you must:

- Put together an accurate and current medical history—a personal health record.
- Maintain complete and honest medication lists for prescription and over-the-counter drugs.
- Follow individualized care plans outlined by your health-care provider, including medication adherence.

- Maintain an accurate record of allergic reactions to food and medicines.
- Understand and own your health-care costs.
- Provide feedback to providers, such as blood sugar and blood pressure daily records.
- Engage in e-mail communications and e-visits instead of always heading to the physician's office or the emergency room or depending upon telephone calls.
- Go online to read test and procedure reports, to do scheduling and referrals, and to educate yourself about various health concerns,
- Work with the medical team to engage in preventive care.
- Do the necessary research on the Internet to understand personal and public health issues.
- Advocate for your own health needs or those of family members; do not wait for the physician to identify those needs.
- Provide a personal health record that ideally links to your physician's electronic medical record.

Patient-Centered Care Alternatives

Retail Clinics

In the ideal health-care environment, you would always go to your primary care office for care. But it is not always possible. Retail clinics, which sprouted in the early days of the twenty-first century, are a good alternative for care when options (other than the emergency room) are not available. These clinics mainly take care of basic health needs. They are set up to provide care on a walk-in basis (no appointment required) during regular hours as well as evening and weekend hours. With the digital tools now available, a summary of everything that occurs during your visit to a retail clinic can be transmitted to your primary care physician. Minor health issues that used to send you to the hospital ER, where the wait is interminable and the cost prohibitive, can be resolved in a retail clinic.

When you visit a retail clinic, you are generally seen by a licensed nurse practitioner who is more than qualified to handle your nonemergency health concerns, such as colds, coughs, ear aches, cuts and bruises, stomach complaints, flu-related symptoms, and strep throat. They can also administer standard flu shots and other injections. Many clinics also offer routine physical exams. Some have expanded their scope of service to include management of chronic conditions or setting of broken bones. Others are conducting smoking cessation programs and counseling related to HIV and STDs. Payers including Aetna, CIGNA, and United Healthcare, and some of the Blues now reimburse for retail clinic visits. Some clinics have a loose affiliation with a local hospital. They are subject to oversight by governmental health agencies, who see that they maintain a level of quality and safety in their practice. Unlike a visit to your doctor, pricing for various services at a retail clinic are posted on a menu board, and if your payer approves the use of the clinic, you just have to make the copayment required. If you need to have a prescription filled, there is usually a pharmacy right there. Retail clinics are also a great option for people who are traveling, fall ill, and can't get in touch with their regular health care provider. If you go to a retail clinic, you must be sure to bring all necessary health information with you, including your medications, health history, and contact information for your regular provider so that you will receive appropriate treatment.

A study by Rand Health showed that a large percentage of people who use retail clinics do not typically have a primary care provider. The population at these clinics tends to be younger patients, minority families, and families with children, often without health insurance. There are very few patients age sixty-five and older. Convenience and low-cost services, short wait times, transparent pricing, and dissatisfaction with existing primary care are the primary reasons study respondents cited for visiting a retail clinic. Many of these patients pay for the retail clinic services out of pocket, and nearly 25 percent of patients who use retail clinics do not have health insurance. The study reported that overall satisfaction with quality of care at the retail clinic is high. In most instances, the retail clinic will refer a patient who needs more complex oversight to a primary care practice or to a hospital.(5)

Community Health Centers

Community health centers (CHCs) and free clinics evolved from President Lyndon Johnson's War on Poverty program, which, in the middle of the 1960s, allocated federal funding for millions of US citizens without health insurance who had great difficulty finding providers to accept them for care. Today, funding for CHCs is tied to several federal and state programs designed to provide health services to underserved populations in both rural and urban areas. Medicaid is the largest source of revenue for CHCs, followed by federal grants. The ambulatory care services offered by these health centers reflect the diverse needs of the population they serve. Generally there is a high demand for gynecologic, family practice, and pediatric services. At the bare minimum, all of the centers offer wellness checkups, immunizations, basic tests, and treatment when you are sick. Many also offer dental care, prescription drugs, and mental health and substance abuse care. The populations served include individuals receiving unemployment benefits, individuals employed in seasonal or part-time work, and those who are experiencing financial hardship and do not have health insurance coverage. Many health centers also offer an array of public services such as translation, transportation, outreach, eligibility assistance, and health education. Community health centers include a large population of young patients who come with a high incidence of chronic conditions like diabetes, asthma, and hypertension in disproportionate numbers to the general population. The centers are often staffed by local physicians, some of whom donate their time. Nurses, nurse practitioners, and lab technicians also staff these facilities. A dispensary is usually located on site where prescriptions are filled. (Narcotic drugs are not available.)

A key provision of the Health Reform Act of 2009 expands the national network of community health centers. The reform legislation increases CHC funding by $11 billion dollars between 2010 and 2015. The legislation includes payment incentives to encourage high quality care and expansion of information technology infrastructure so that these centers can serve as patient-centered medical homes. Multiple studies have documented health centers' efficacy in reducing the delivery of low-birth-weight babies and reducing the number of hospitalizations for patients with chronic conditions. Approximately one-third of health centers in the United States are accredited by the Joint Commission on Accreditation of Healthcare Organizations (JCAHO), a private not-for-profit organization that operates accreditation programs for hospitals and other health-care organizations throughout the United States. JCAHO sets the standards of care to which health-care organizations aspire. A majority of state governments have come to recognize JCAHO accreditation as a condition of licensure and therefore permit the receipt of Medicaid reimbursement at those locations.

A Commonwealth Fund survey of community health centers found that the more medical home characteristics a center possessed, the more likely it is to report better communication and coordination with specialty care providers and local hospitals. The study further indicated that 40 percent of health centers use electronic medical records, which is nearly the same rate as practitioners throughout the country. Fifty-seven percent of centers reported they electronically access patients' laboratory tests results on a routine basis, and 45 percent routinely order laboratory tests electronically. The report found that enhancing a center's use of health IT is related to better coordinated patient care. (6)

For nearly thirty years, a community health center located in downtown Sioux Falls, South Dakota, has seen thousands of patients from a variety of backgrounds and nationalities, including underserved individuals who have lived in the area for many years and an influx of refugees from countries throughout the world who recently migrated to this region as a part of the refugee resettlement program sponsored by the US Department of Health and Human Services. The Sioux Falls Community Health Center is a large-scale operation that includes family practice clinics, mental health services, pediatric services, and a Ryan White early intervention program for HIV and AIDS patients, as well as dental and vision services. Interpreters are available for patients who have little or no English skills. The staff also includes nurse case managers and social workers who counsel patients and educate them in health management and prevention, and a volunteer cardiologist and dermatologist.

According to Katie Wick, Clinical Services Manager, the Sioux Falls Community Health Center in 2009 served over 12,200 patients who had over 40,000 visits, of which 28 percent were pediatric visits. The number one diagnosis that the clinic addresses is depression, for which they have counselors and a psychiatrist available. There is also a high percentage of treatment for diabetes and cardiovascular disease. The dental clinic is staffed by three dentists. In partnership with the local Lions Club, they also offer eye exams. They even have vans that go out into the streets of Sioux Falls to pick up homeless people and drive them to the center for treatment. With or without health insurance, everyone who comes to the Sioux Falls Community Health

Center is treated. Over 50 percent of patients do not have health insurance or are underinsured; the other 50 percent have Medicaid, Medicare, or a private health plan. Patients have to pay a minimum of fifteen dollars for a medical visit and thirty-five dollars for a dental visit. A sliding fee structure is offset by federal grants. Many patients are homeless or in transition.

The major issues for the health center are having enough providers to treat all the patients who come to them and educating patients to think about their health before there is a crisis. They are also outgrowing their current space and recently added three new exam rooms. The Sioux Falls Community Health Center includes two satellite clinics located in the public schools, where they provide general health services, flu shots, and other inoculations. Although they may not meet all of the "official" requirements of a patient-centered medical home, to the over twelve thousand individuals that they serve, the Sioux Falls Community Health Center is their medical home, and they come back again and again for medical care and services that go above and beyond basic medical needs. (7)

E-visits

Online health consultations, or e-visits, enable you and your physicians to connect on the Internet using a secure portal site to address nonemergency issues and important questions you may have. They help maintain a continuum of care. Messaging software enables you to log into a secure website and fill out templates and logic-based questions, which are sent to a physician who will answer your communication and engage in a dialogue with you asynchronously. You may send a request for an e-visit, and it can take twenty-four hours, or as much as seventy-two hours on a weekend, for a response.

The benefit of an e-visit is that it saves you time and money, since you do not have to travel to see your doctor in person. Make no mistake about it—the e-visit does not replace your face-to-face visit with your doctor for more important and comprehensive medical issues. E-visits should be used for only minor ailments such as colds and sore throats, rashes, or bruises. You might also request an e-visit in instances where you can send a digital photo ahead for discussion or for a periodic review of a chronic condition. It is also an efficient way to have a general follow-up consultation with your doctor in between visits. A growing number of health plans, including Aetna and Cigna, have begun to pay doctors for online visits with their patients.

E-visits should be based on personal interaction with your provider and should occur only when you and your physician have a preexisting relationship that includes a face-to-face encounter within the current year. Unfortunately, many patients use this technology for online medical consultations at one of the hundreds of websites that offer free or nominally priced medical consults with doctors you have never met. These consultations are priced at between twenty-five and forty dollars—the approximate amount that you might typically be charged for co-pay for a regular office visit. The medical professionals who are talking to you at these sites have no reference points regarding your medical history. Although you can get quick answers, the individuals you are talking with could misinterpret your problem or make erroneous conclusions because they are not familiar with your specific case. People surfing the Internet for health information admittedly often do not check the source and date of the health information they are reading. Engaging in an e-visit with a physician who does not have access to your health record and whom you have never met is not wise. The American Academy of Family Physicians states on their website that they support enhanced-access physician-patient interactions, including virtual/electronic visits or "e-visits," that occur over safe, secure, online communication systems. Their guidelines for e-visits include the following: (8)

- E-visits should be used only when you have an established relationship with your provider.
- The patient initiates the process and agrees to e-visit service terms, privacy policy, and charge for receiving asynchronous care from a physician or other qualified health professional.
- Electronic communication occurs over a HIPAA-compliant online connection.
- An e-visit includes the total interchange of online inquiries and other communications associated with this single patient encounter.
- The physician appropriately documents the e-visits, including all pertinent communication related to the encounter, in the patient's medical/health record.

- The physician or other qualified health professional has a defined period of time within which responses to an e-visit request are completed.
- E-visits should be a payable physician service.

The Henry Ford Medical Group of the Henry Ford Hospital is a part of the world-renowned Henry Ford Health System located on West Grand Boulevard in the New Center area of Detroit. It is one of the nation's largest group practices, with over one thousand physicians and researchers in more than forty specialties. Henry Ford offers e-visits to their patients. To initiate an e-visit, patients go online to their portal (MyHealth) at www.henryford.com and login to their secure page. They have two options:

1. *Describe their nonurgent health and medical issues to their primary care provider. Based upon their question, a series of queries will be posted to the patient; subsequent questions are based on their responses. The branching logic in the interviews provides physicians with the information they need to assess the patient.*
2. *Describe their nonhealth issues in a preset series of questions around the following chronic conditions: diabetes, hypertension, depression, asthma, and coronary artery disease.*

Henry Ford physicians can respond to both types of visits in a number of ways: by ordering lab tests, changing or ordering new prescriptions, instructing the patient to take action at home, or advising him or her to come into the office. Each e-visit costs twenty dollars. Patients are not charged if their issue is not resolved and an office visit is necessary.

Initially, the program designers thought that people were going to use e-visits for low-acuity health problems; however, their experience with the e-visits proved otherwise. Physicians in the system found e-visits to be most helpful for those patients suffering from chronic conditions because it enabled primary care physicians to make more frequent adjustments to their patient's treatment regimen and achieve better clinical goals between office visits. Henry Ford also thought young people would flock to this program because they tend to be online more, but that did not prove to be the case either. Instead they found the average age of the e-visit user was forty-four to fifty-one years and a person who suffers from a chronic condition. Henry Ford also realized that e-visits have a number of benefits, including enhancing patient and physician communication.

E-visits elicit the highest satisfaction scores from patients and from physicians. Most importantly, the people who have e-visits take better care of themselves overall, as evidenced by their HEDIS scores (Health Effectiveness Data and Information Set), a widely used measurement to determine performance in the managed health environment. Patients using e-visits improved in every measure and became more engaged and involved with their care. (9)

A CMS ruling established in 2009 now allows physicians to bill Medicare for electronic consultations (e-visits) following inpatient visits. It also adds new codes specifically for telemedicine consultations for health-care providers who are consulted by a patient's physician but are not available for in-person consultations. These e-visits, performed in real time with interactive communications systems, are for the purpose of monitoring a patient's progress, recommending care-management changes, or providing a new plan of care. Once CMS makes the e-visit a standard, reimbursed part of payment to physicians, most payers will follow.

RelayHealth, an online communication and connectivity solution, pioneered the e-visit. Launched in 1999, RelayHealth of Atlanta, which is now part of McKesson Corporation, provides secure, web-enabled communications that offer patients webVisit consultations, prescription refills and renewals, results delivery, requests for appointment scheduling and referrals, health education information, and more. RelayHealth's webVisit is a clinically structured web-based interview to communicate nonurgent routine symptoms to a physician. Created by clinicians for handling online clinical questions, the formalized questionnaire invites patients to choose from a menu of symptoms and answer a series of questions related to that specific condition. The physician is presented with the full information and subsequently is able to make informed quality care decisions. The doctor can respond to a RelayHealth online visit by phone or if necessary request an in-office visit. The RelayHealth system checks the patient's insurance eligibility during the webVisit, sends a claim to the health plan for reimbursement, collects the co-pay, and sends it to the physician. Many companies are now offering e-visits for their employees using RelayHealth or other services. (10)

American Well takes online communication between you and your physicians to the next level, offering real-time consults on any aspect of medicine, with qualified, credentialed physicians. These online interactions are available through a health plan, although you can use the system independently through local operators in your state if your health plan doesn't offer the service. The American Well system allows physicians (and other health-care providers) to make themselves available at a convenient time and enables you to select a doctor or specialty that can address your immediate concern. All that is needed is a working online connection and a browser, or a regular telephone. Once you request a session with a physician, you can choose to engage in an interactive discussion to supply your health history. Alternatively, through integration with other online systems, American Well can gather your health history, lab data, personal health record, and other relevant material. The goal is to be sure that the physician talking with you has your complete health profile. The average time for an American Well online consult is ten minutes, with the option to extend the encounter if needed. The visit's total cost (a portion of which may be covered by your health plan) is typically thirty-five to forty-five dollars—a lot less expensive and a lot more convenient than sending you to a medical center to see a high-level specialist in person.

At the end of the encounter, both you and your physician have complete documentation of the visit, which is stored securely in an archive online and is available to you and your other providers for future reference. Recommended follow-up and referrals are built into the system so you know if you need additional tests or other actions. It is up to you to follow through. Additionally, a full transcript of the conversation can be transmitted to your PCP, if you choose. Several payer companies are now offering online care services using American Well technology, including Blue Cross Blue Shield of Hawaii, Blue Cross Blue Shield of Minnesota, OptumHealth (a business of UnitedHealth Group), TriWest Healthcare Alliance, Blue Cross Blue Shield of Western New York, Blue Shield of Northeastern New York, Ascension Health, Rite Aid pharmacy, and WellPoint. (11)

A Forrester Research study that looked at interactions between patients and care professional that occur online and what users are generally doing online found that over 50 percent of those individuals who engage in e-visits also have researched a specific medical condition online, and over 40 percent have researched a specific medication. This mail survey conducted in 2009 involved more than five thousand individuals who live in North America. (12)

**Percentage of consumers who have performed the following
activities ONLINE in the past 12 months**

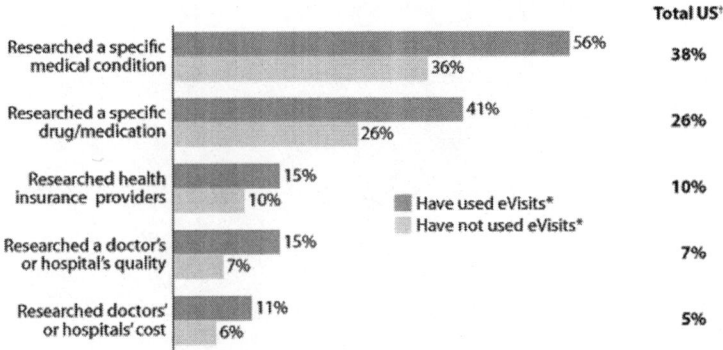

Total US[†]

		Total US[†]
Researched a specific medical condition	56% / 36%	38%
Researched a specific drug/medication	41% / 26%	26%
Researched health insurance providers	15% / 10%	10%
Researched a doctor's or hospital's quality	15% / 7%	7%
Researched doctors' or hospitals' cost	11% / 6%	5%

■ Have used eVisits*
■ Have not used eVisits*

*Base: US consumers whose primary doctor offers eVisits
†Base: US consumers

Source: North American Technographics® Media, Marketing, Consumer Technology, And Healthcare Benchmark Survey, Q3 2009 (US, Canada)

57094   Source: Forrester Research, Inc.

House Calls

In an era when many patients complain about paying too much money for too little time with their doctors, Dr. Susan Rutten Wasson, who is trained as an internist and pediatrician, has a different approach that is as close to patient-centered care as you can get. Dr. Wasson, who has been in practice for ten years, sees patients by appointment in her small town office in Osakis, Minnesota. She allows her patients same-day scheduling for office visits and spends at least a half hour with each patient, for which she charges a fifty-dollar cash fee out of pocket. Dr. Wasson accepts no insurance and thus is not bogged down with billing third-party payers. Prior to opening her office in Osakis, Dr. Wasson's practice consisted primarily of house calls. She still makes some house calls today to help patients who have difficulty getting to her office.

"You learn a lot about people when you see where and how they live," she says. Dr. Wasson does not schedule regular visits; her patients come to see her when they need to, although she does see individuals with chronic conditions at least once a year. In a typical visit, Dr. Wasson will check blood pressure, weight, and other vitals and talk with her patients in detail about what is bothering them. She sends her patients to a local clinic to have blood drawn and refers her seriously ill patients to one of the local hospitals or to the major medical centers

in either the Twin Cities; Fargo, North Dakota; or Sioux Falls, South Dakota; or she sends them to the Mayo Clinic. Most of the individuals she serves are what she calls "good country people" who make their living by farming or trucking. Many of them have never used a computer, cell phone, or e-mail and have no access to technology. English is a second language for many patients, and computers are not an option.

Dr. Wasson is a firm believer that people must take responsibility for their own health, but she clearly guides them in making decisions. She follows the tenets she learned in medical school to run through a list of possibilities and to examine her patients carefully and narrow down the possibilities. "Too many tests," she says, "get ordered in a shotgun approach." She believes in sending her patients for tests (e.g., CAT scans, MRIs, X-rays, or extensive blood work) only when the visual diagnosis is unclear. She is convinced that people in general have no idea of what these procedures cost until they see a bill. Patients hear about Dr. Wasson from the local pharmacist and from other patients. Many come to her for a second opinion. She is always busy.

Several physicians and physician groups are once again making house calls to home-bound patients who cannot get to the doctor's office. This represents the very definition of patient-centered care. Today's physicians who do home visits can not only do a thorough physical exam, but can perform EKG testing, draw blood, and even do an X-ray using the latest digital machinery, which is portable and efficient. Furthermore, with electronic records, they can record all of their test results and observations right on a laptop for communication to various entities, including hospitals, payers, and other doctors or specialists you might see. According to the American Medical Association (AMA), six million Americans receive medical care at home. A study in the Archives of Internal Medicine found that 65 percent of family doctors and 44 percent of all internists reported that they might make house calls.

New York City's Presbyterian/Weill Cornell Medical Center has sponsored a program called "House Calls" since 1977 to meet the needs of a portion of the elderly home-bound city population who can no longer navigate their way to their doctor. The program serves over seventy households in neighborhoods around the hospital and enables the doctors in the program to spend quality time with their patients and get to know them well. (13)

Microsoft has brought back the old-fashioned doctor's house call for employees in a bid to slash costs, improve employee health, and contain potential pandemics. Microsoft is one of the only employers, and by far the largest, offering such personalized health services to workers. Their house call program, called Mobile Medicine, got its start in 2006 after a massive analysis of the company's health-care data revealed that their employees, like others, were using the emergency room mostly for non-life-threatening, problems such as ear infections, skeletal bruises, and the flu. Such trips to the emergency room average $1,500–$2,000 a visit, according to the American Academy of Home Care Physicians. As a result, Microsoft's policy of having family doctors show up at their employee's bedsides, sometimes in the dead of night, makes economic sense. Microsoft's data claims that they have reduced health-care costs by approximately 35 percent with the house call program. Additionally, the company claims that the strategy gives primary care doctors more responsibility to manage patients' treatments and keep employees healthier in the long term. (14)

Why Patient-Centered Care?

As an e-patient, your goal has to be focused on insuring that you are receiving the best care that current technology and the trained medical professional has to offer you, within a reasonable health-care budget. That is why you must accept the care of trained nurse practitioners and physician assistants when a qualified primary care physician is not available. It is why you should find yourself a medical home where your basic health needs can be met. It is why, when you are stymied by the system, you can with assurance turn to a retail clinic or a community health center for care. It is why you advocate for your primary care providers to create the secure web portals that enable you to engage in web visits and access information that puts you in control of managing your care. It is going to take an enormous clamor from patients to insure that patient-centered care becomes and remains a top priority for the medical establishment. At the end of the day, patient-centered care and the medical home will bring about reforms both in terms of financial management and in quality of care. It will encourage the spread of participatory medicine that is critical to resolving some of the issues regarding fair and equitable health care for all citizens.

Dell published a survey in 2010 that polled 50 hospital executives and 309 patients who had recently been in the hospital as patients. The patients universally embraced the idea of advanced health information technology. Among the obvious requests for better food, lower costs, and more nurses, over 80 percent were looking for better communication with their providers and more accurate recordkeeping. This bar chart outlines in detail what patients want, and it is obvious from the results they are seeking technologies that would make their medical delivery more collaborative and patient-centered. One of the survey questions was: As you consider how care providers help you manage your personal wellness and care, do you agree or disagree that each of the flowing capabilities or tools should be implemented to improve your patient experience? (15)

What Patients Want
% Responding Somewhat or Strongly Agree

- Electronic Access to information about a hospital (medical expertise, physician experience, insurance acceptance, etc.) to help you determine which hospital to visit — **81%**
- Electronic prescription processing to allow health care providers and pharmacies to communicate without paper — **76%**
- Making it possible for EHRs to be shared between your physician, hospital, rehab center, laboratory etc. — **74%**
- Providing more information electronically, such as access to discharge and follow-up care instructions after a hospital stay. — **73%**
- Email access to your doctor so you can ask questions and discuss your health via electronic mail — **71%**
- Implementing EHRs — **69%**
- Hospitals and physicians publishing their quality rankings on their website for your review and consideration — **67%**
- Independent third party internet portals where patients can rate their experiences with doctors, hospitals and clinics (not sponsored by a physician or physician's office) — **65%**
- New technologies that enable your physician to remotely monitor your wellness by checking your vital statistics and treatment response (e.g. blood pressure) from a device you use in your home — **64%**
- Introducing more tele-medicine capabilities so that you can meet with your physician to discuss health issues over the Internet or telephone — **62%**
- Providing access to your personal health records through an Internet portal or private website — **61%**
- Providing check-in or admission kiosks at hospital and physician facilities — **60%**
- Technologies that allow your insurance company to remotely track vital statistics and treatment response to help you manage your prescriptions and help you manage a chronic disease — **48%**

Survey Question: *As you consider how care providers help you manage your personal wellness and care, do you agree or disagree that each of the following new capabilities or tools should be implemented to improve your patient experience?*

From the Dell Executive and Patient Survey. Reprinted with permission from Dell © 2011.

Key Points

1. We are moving to a patient-centered model of care that creates a care team including the individual, the health-care professionals, the family, and all others who may be involved with the individual's care, including social workers and therapists. Shared responsibility by this collaborative team in a patient-centered medical home will insure that you will experience the safe, high-quality, continuous care that you deserve.
2. Digital communication technology, including the Internet, secure portals, e-mail, e-visits, and smartphones, are critical components of the medical home.
3. Physician assistants and nurse practitioners will fill in the personnel gap created by a critical shortage of primary care physicians. They will serve as the primary caretakers for individuals who are triaged to doctors when needed.
4. Retail clinics are spreading throughout the country and provide alternative care models for individuals who need immediate care when their medical home is not available.
5. Community health centers provide medical homes for the uninsured, the poor, and those who cannot access care via their workplace and health insurers.
6. E-visits, which are being reimbursed by some payers including Medicare, supplement office visits for nonurgent medical issues and the management of chronic conditions.
7. House calls are becoming more commonplace, especially in the inner city where elderly and disabled patients are not able to get to the doctor's office or a health center, or in rural locations where patients cannot travel the distances required to see the doctor.

Notes

1. National Academy of Sciences, "Formulating New Rules to Redesign and Improve Care," *Crossing the Quality Chasm,* National Academy of Sciences, 2001, p. 61.

2. A. Milstein and E. Gilbertson, "American Medical Home Runs," *Health Affairs,* Millwood, 28(5)(2009): 1317–26; doi:10.1377/hlthaff.28.5.1317.

3. Policy statement, "The Medical Home," *Pediatrics,* 110(2002):184–186, http://www.aappolicy/aappolicy.org, http://www.aap.org/healthtopics/medicalhome.html

4. Patient Centered Primary Care Collaborative, "Patient Centered Medical Home: Building Evidence and Momentum: A Compilation of PCMH Pilot and Demonstration Projects," PCPCC, 2008, pp. 51–53, http://www.pcpcc.net.

5. Ateev Mehrotra, MD; Hagnsheng Liu, PhD; John L. Adams, PhD; et al., "Comparing Costs and Quality of Care at Retail Clinics with That of Other Medical Settings for Three Common Illnesses," *Rand Health,* 2010.

6. Meredith B. Rosenthal, PhD; Howard B. Beckman, MD; et al., "Will the Patient-Centered Medical Home Improve Efficiency and Reduce Costs of Care? A Measurement and Research Agenda," *Medical Care Research and Review,* August 2010, 67(4):476–84.

7. Katie Wick, Clinical Services Manager, Sioux Falls Community Health Center, in an interview with the author.

8. The American Academy of Family Physicians (AAFP) Guidelines for E-visits, http://www.aafp.org/online/en/home/policy/policies/e/evisits.html.

9. Pamela Landis, Director of Information Technology at Henry Ford Health Systems, in communication with the author.

10. www.relayhealth.com

11. www.americanwell.com

12. Elizabeth Boehm, "Which Consumers Are Healthcare eVisit Early Adopters," *Forrester Research,* June 3, 2010.

13. ew York-Presbyterian, "House Calls Program at New York-Presbyterian/Weill Cornell Helps City's Elderly," New York-Presbyterian, Dec 16, 2003, http://www.nyp.org/news/hospital/house-calls.html.

14. Michelle Conlin, "Companies Eager to Cut Health-Care Costs May Do Well to Consider the Home Doctor Visits Microsoft Offers," *Bloomberg Business Week,* Management and Leadership, November 5, 2009, 5:00 p.m. EST.

15. The Dell Executive and Patient Survey, 2010, Page 5.

Chapter Eight

Web Resources

Advances in computer technology and the Internet have changed the way America works, learns, and communicates. The Internet has become an integral part of America's economic, political, and social life.

President William J. Clinton, President of the United States (1993–2001)

Health Care Finds the Internet

The Internet, which was the creation of scientists and US military specialists, now gives you instant, efficient communications that can transmit your information in nano-seconds. Built on a philosophy of openness and bound together by an endless infrastructure of digital connections, the Internet allows you to ship the entire collected works of Shakespeare across the Worldwide Web in the blink of an eye.

Today, your personal health-care information, which used to be the exclusive province of a health-care professional, is available to you on the Internet twenty-four-seven, if you choose to store it that way. With the spread of wireless technology, you can access that information not only from a desktop PC but from a wireless laptop, from a handheld device, and from your smartphone. You can also find important, relevant answers to your health questions, access independent medical diagnosis, contract health services, and make connections with individuals who suffer from similar health problems.

A young woman living in Oregon gave birth to a premature baby girl who had lung issues that could cause brain damage. The woman and her husband were devastated. Their doctors and nurses, although caring, competent, and sympathetic, were not able to give them a lot of hope or much information. In desperation, the woman and her husband turned to the Internet, and they found web communities where they connected with other couples who had premature infants with similar conditions. Although the Internet did not offer a magic formula for curing their baby, the web offered them hope as well as suggestions about new tests and drugs, which they were able to discuss with their medical providers and take advantage of to find a remedy for their baby, who fortunately responded well and got better.

The Pew Research Center (Pew Internet and American Life Project) is an independent opinion research group that focuses on media and public policy. They conduct studies on the behavior of the American public and the Internet. In April 2009 they released a definitive study, *Social Life of Health Information,* which looked at how the American public used the Internet to find health information. The research was based on data from telephone interviews conducted by Princeton Survey Research Associates between November 19 and December 20, 2008, among a national sample of 2,253 adults. The results indicated that in 2008, 74 percent of American adults were online, and 61 percent of those adults look online for health information. This represents a significant change since the Pew Internet research conducted in the spring of 2000, when 46 percent of American adults had access to the Internet, and 25 percent looked online for health information. Other interesting results of this study revealed that:

- 52 percent of all online health inquiries are on behalf of someone other than the person typing in the search terms
- 41 percent of people looking for health information have read someone else's commentary or experience about health or medical issues on an online news group, website, or blog.
- 24 percent consulted rankings or reviews online of doctors or other providers.

- 24 percent consulted rankings or reviews online of hospitals or other medical facilities.
- 19 percent signed up to receive updates about health or medical issues.

Despite the increasing popularity of social network sites and status update services, few people in 2008 used them to gather and share health information.(1)

In 2011, Pew conducted another study, *Health Topics*, on the uses of the Internet for gathering health-care information. This study revealed that of 80 percent of Internet users now look online for health information, making health care the third most popular online pursuit. This report is also based in part on a national telephone survey conducted by Princeton Survey Research Associates International that included 3,001 adults.

A profile of some of the topics that most interest these Internet health information seekers in 2011 include:
- 66 percent look online for information about a specific disease or medical problem.
- 56 percent look online for information about a certain medical treatment or procedure.
- 44 percent look online for information about doctors or other health professionals.
- 36 percent look online for information about hospitals or other medical facilities
- 33 percent look online for information related to health insurance, including private insurance, Medicare, or Medicaid.

About six in ten say their Internet searches have an impact on their own health or the way they care for someone else. Sixty percent say the information found online affected a decision about how to treat an illness or, condition and 50 percent indicated that their online searches have changed their overall approach to maintaining their health or the health of someone they care for.(2)

Clearly the Internet now attracts an increasing number of people who are seeking answers that they are not finding using other sources, including their health-care providers. On any given day, there are more people online seeking medical advice than actually visit health professionals. These individuals search for health information, research a diagnosis or prescription, prepare for surgery, find out how to best recover from an illness, or seek emotional support for a unique problem. Although the first and foremost source of information on your health should always be your primary care physician, there is a lot to be gained by supplementing your understanding of health issues by checking credible Internet resources and connecting with others. Online support groups provide a particularly valuable asset. Finding individuals with the same or similar conditions who can help you understand all of your options could make a significant difference in your eventual outcome. Today, there is a website for virtually every specific disease or problem, where you can find detailed information that outlines treatment options and connects you with people who understand what you are going through. You merely have to type the name of the disease in your browser window and chances are, you will find a group to talk with.

Ken was diagnosed with fibromyalgia (FM) in 1996, following twelve years of searching for answers about why he had periods of numbness in his extremities and flu-like symptoms. After finally receiving the diagnosis, he found that his doctors had little to offer him by way of remedies or ideas on how to treat the disease.

Ken and his wife, Donna, began searching the Internet for information from their home in Regina, Saskatchewan. In 1996, there was not much available regarding FM. They found scattered bits and pieces of information, but nothing comprehensive. They decided to put together what they had collected and create a website that they called "Fibrohugs." Soon they began to get e-mails from people all over the world thanking them for developing the website. They set up message-board forums and later added a live chat room. The twenty to twenty-five people who gathered at Fibrohugs to chat on a regular basis began to feel like a little family. Over time, doctors recommended the site to their patients. By the end of 2009, the site had nearly twenty-seven thousand members, and over four hundred million individuals had visited Fibrohugs. Five to ten new people join as members every day.

About three years ago, when a family member of Ken's developed cancer, Ken and Donna discovered there was a serious lack of one-on-one personal support available for cancer patients. They launched a sister site to Fibrohugs called Cancer Hugs. Ironically, four months into building the site, Donna was diagnosed with cancer. The Fibrohugs family suffered with them, encouraged them, and mourned with Ken when, sadly, Donna passed away. (3)

Information Access

Ben was diagnosed with prostate cancer. The treatment options for his particular form of cancer were thoroughly explained by his doctors, in whom he had confidence, but even with a second opinion consult, he was confused as to which way to turn. He had to decide among the choices: watch and wait (to see if the tumor grows larger), radiation therapy, radiation followed by surgery, surgery alone, or hormone treatment. To add to his confusion, there are different surgical approaches, some of which are more invasive with more potential aftereffects than others. His doctors could not tell him which option might be better. Ben turned to the Internet and went to several cancer sites, joined chat rooms and discussion groups, and talked with people who had been in the same circumstances and who could relay their experiences. He not only found details about other people's treatments, but lots of support and comfort. He was able to make a decision based upon his own research and knowledge.

The sheer volume of health information on the Internet changes the dynamic of health information dissemination. At the beginning of 2009, there were approximately 170 million websites on the Internet and 70 million blogs. Of those, several million websites and more than one million blogs dealt with health-related information. These sites include health content that provides you with information for staying well, for preventing and managing disease, and for making decisions about health, health care, health products, or health services, as well as information that can help you avoid a major medical error or misdiagnosis.

At age fifty-two, Trisha found a large lump on her torso. She immediately saw her primary care physician, who sent her to a surgeon who removed the lump and sent it out for diagnosis. More than two anxious weeks went by before Trisha heard back from the surgeon, who finally told her that she had a very rare form of cancer for which there was no cure. The surgeon explained that with chemotherapy, she might gain two years of life. Trisha immediately accessed the Internet for information while she waited to see an oncologist, who was not much more encouraging than the surgeon.

However, the oncologist did send Trisha for blood work and a CT scan. Both came back negative for any abnormalities. Trisha was feeling fine; with the mixed the test results, she suspected pieces were missing. While waiting to see the next doctor, she continued to search the Internet for help interpreting her tests. By the time she saw the second oncologist, she was empowered with all the necessary information. This doctor agreed that there were significant doubts about her diagnosis and, with her permission, sent the test results to the National Institutes of Health. Three weeks later, she received a notice that, indeed, she did not have the cancer.

Trisha went through an agonizing period. Because she is an e-patient who persisted in searching for every possible clue and learning about the experiences and opinions of others, Trisha was able to avert an alarming misdiagnosis that could have led to unpleasant and risky chemotherapy and even death. Although Trisha's web searches did not provide absolute answers, the information she found set up enough red flags to make her suspicious and able to convince the second oncologist to pursue the issue. This approach turned out to be exactly correct.

Information Overload

Information access is a good thing because it insures that you will be a more informed, health-care-literate patient who can participate completely in taking care of yourself and your family. However, the sheer amount of health-related information present on the Internet and in the media puts you in extreme overload. As a result, it is difficult to filter what is credible and reliable and what is hype. Below are guidelines regarding what to look for on websites that you can rely on to provide you with the health-care information you need.

1. Questions to Ask
- Who developed this site? Is the author or authors clearly identified? Are the credentials of the author listed?

- Does the page show when it was last updated? Are the links to other resources still active?
- Is contact information provided so that you can e-mail, call, or write the web sponsor?
- What is the purpose of the information?
- Can the information be verified in other sources?

2. Use trustworthy websites of established health-care organizations.

- Websites ending in .gov sponsored by federal, state, or local governments or reputable government agencies (e.g., HHS, CDC, and NIH), which can be held to the test for accuracy, reliability, and impartiality.
- Sites of the major medical institutions (e.g., Johns Hopkins Medical Center, Partners, Kaiser Permanente, and Mayo Clinic).
- Websites of organizations that are focused on specific diseases, such as the American Cancer Society, American Lung Association, and the Brain Tumor Society, are excellent resources for information on these conditions and also a great place to find individuals who are experiencing similar problems with whom you can interact. These sites have a vested interested in helping you and your physicians find information of value.

3. Check seals of approval that insure credibility and reliability of information.

- **Health-on-the-Net Foundation (HON)** is a nongovernmental nonprofit foundation supported by the United Nations Economic and Social Council and designed to guide consumers to reliable, credible health and medical information on the Internet.
- **Hi-Ethics, Inc., or Health Internet Ethics,** unites the most widely used health Internet sites supporting high ethical standards. Member companies are committed to earning the trust and confidence of consumers who choose to use Internet health services for improving their health and health care.
- **Internet Healthcare Coalition (IHCC)** is an independent and nonindustry aligned group dedicated to educating health-care consumers, professionals, educators, marketers, and public

policymakers on the full range of uses of the Internet to deliver high-quality health-care information and services.

4 Sites to Avoid

- Websites that offer suspicious remedies that promise fast weight loss, instant hair replacement, miracle cures, nutritional supplements, great healing.
- Websites that advertise doctors who will supply a quick fix.
- Websites that are filled with medical jargon.
- Websites that try to sell you products, vitamins, health services, common drugs, or herbal remedies.
- Websites that are overly negative about traditional treatment.

Reputable websites require that you have a prescription written by your health provider. They strictly obey the regulations enforced by US government agencies. Many sites on the web that sell you drugs were developed outside the United States where there is no federal agency such as the FDA monitoring the research and distribution of drugs.

A study reported in the Journal of the American Medical Association (September 17, 2003) reviewed 443 websites that contained information on eight best-selling herbal products. Researchers found that many sites were selling the supplements, and over half of these contained illegal and misleading claims that their products can treat, prevent, diagnose, or cure specific diseases. Many of the websites analyzed contained illegal health claims and information that could potentially harm. What was more alarming about the findings is that more than half of the respondent Internet users reported that they thought "almost all" of the health information they encountered on the Internet was credible.

Good websites state their purpose on the home page and include site maps and search options for easy navigation. Always check to see that the information is current. You want to find sites that focus on content that meets your specific needs. Many sites include chat rooms and message boards where you can post your questions and share personal information that can be valuable.

Best Websites

Consumer Information Services

General health and wellness websites are the most familiar and frequently used sites for e-Patients. Many target a specific population such as women's or men's health, cancer patients, children's health, etc. Others have a broader, more comprehensive perspective, for example Yahoo Health, WebMD, and Mayo Clinic, as well as MSN search, Google, or Bing, where you can search any health topic and hundreds of websites and blogs will come up. With so many websites and blogs that deal with health-care issues relevant to consumers, many of them written by experts in the health-care field, you are probably asking yourself, how does one filter through this tower of Babel?

A good starting point for the consumer to begin a web health search is from a gateway website such as the federal government's Healthfinder www.healthfinder.gov NOAH www.noahhealth.org a New York-based group of health and science libraries; or www.health.gov, a site that links to many government-initiated sites to identify general health information resources, government agencies, and current health news releases. Other gateways include www.medlineplus.gov from the National Library of Medicine and the National Institutes of Health, where you and your physicians can find information on virtually every facet of medicine and alternative medicine consisting of seven hundred topics based upon reliable medically approved information, including a database of doctors, dentists, hospitals, and clinics, and an online directory of drugs and herbal supplements.

Not all of the links that come up from a search on these sites are as reliable as they should be. To distinguish those that contain good health information from those that are questionable, check the site sponsor, the information offered, and the currency of the information and the credibility of the information source.

The Medical Library Association has released a top-ten list of most useful websites (www.mlanet.org/resources/medspeak/top ten.htm):
- Cancer.gov

- Centers for Disease Control and Prevention (CDC)
- familydoctor.org
- Healthfinder.com
- HIVInSite.com
- Kidshealth.com
- Mayo Clinic.com
- MEDEM: an information partnership of medical societies
- MEDLINE plus (English | Spanish)
- NOAH: New York Online Access to Health

Descriptions for each of these sites and other valuable consumer health information resources are as follows (those with * indicate the top ten).

Gateway Sites

www.healthfinder.gov

Healthfinder links to a broad range of consumer health and human service information resources. Healthfinder was developed and is maintained by the US Department of Health and Human Services. It allows you to submit web searches for medical, pharmaceutical, or health-care information and receive targeted useful health information free of charge. This gateway website links to selected online publications, clearinghouses, databases, and over 1,500 websites. It provides information on every conceivable health topic.

www.google.com/Top/Health/

The Google search engine is based on the Open Directory Project (DMOZ, directory.mozilla.org) and is a multilingual, open-content directory of web links that are maintained by a community of volunteer editors who keep the content up to date and relevant. The search engine includes Harvard Medical School's consumer health information and journal databases and a complete spectrum of health topics for individuals of all ages. Subject covered include: men and women's health, conditions and diseases, health research, informatics, and general consumer health concerns such as weight loss, travel health, nutrition, insurance issues, fitness, cosmetic surgery, medications, and many more.

www.yahoohealth.com

This website is a compendium of everyday health and wellness topics including diseases, conditions, fitness, nutrition, and articles and advice on health issues written for the consumer. There is significant overlap between Google Health and Yahoo Health.

www.noahhealth.org

This site is sponsored by a New York-based group of health and science libraries. It is written in both English and Spanish languages and provides four thousand health/science information links on every topic.

www.medlineplus.gov

This portal site, sponsored by US Federal Government branches including the National Library of Medicine and the National Institutes of Health, is based upon reliable, medically approved information. Over three thousand doctors, nurse practitioners, and editors contribute content to Medline plus, which is available in both English and Spanish versions. It includes photo illustrations an extensive drug database and over four thousand articles about disease, tests, and symptoms, as well as a medical encyclopedia and a database of doctors, dentists, and hospitals, and clinics. The Medline plus online directory of drugs also includes a database on herbal supplements. The entire site is a great resource for the health-care professional; however, portions of this site could be technical.

www.cdc.gov

This website was developed by the Center for Disease Control (CDC) to provide all of the stakeholders in health care with information on public health issues. One of the mandates for the CDC is to maintain communications with state and local government agencies, federal government partners, and the general public. The website is the major communication channel to accomplish this and includes travel alerts, vaccine requirements, food and beverage, swimming and insect warnings, and disease outbreaks. The CDC website also sponsors podcasts and publications. Discrete sections of information on the site are specifically targeted to consumers. The CDC's specific formats for communication enables it to provide the appropriate assistance and information to the general public.

General Health and Wellness

www.familydoctor.org

This site from the American Academy of Family Physicians features comprehensive consumer health information in both English and Spanish. Some of its interesting features include the "Smart Patient Guide" to help you advocate for your own health care; a guide to over-the-counter medications; a list of parameters to help you choose a family doctor; and Health Tools, a section that takes you to links on conditions from A to Z, with search by symptom and disease. At www.familydoctor.org, you can also find answers to insurance questions, Medicare Part D, and other public policy issues. There is a link titled "Advocacy" that enables you to send messages to Congress on health-care issues you are concerned about.

www.yourdiseaserisk.com

This site provides you with information on disease prevention and ranks your personal risk for five diseases: cancer, diabetes, heart attack, stroke and osteoporosis. It includes an interactive tool that measures your risk of these diseases by asking a set of questions to come up with the risk possibility. The site also provides you with personalized tips for prevention.

www.nccam.nih.gov\

This is the website for the National Center for Complementary and Alternative Medicine, a subdivision of the National Institutes of Health. It includes important information about the benefits and risks of complementary and alternative medicine, with an A-Z index of health topics. It also contains research-based information on many alternative medicine solutions, including acupuncture, herbal remedies, gingko, probiotics, and St. John's wort; warnings about health fraud; and advice on how to deal your health insurer as related to alternative medicine.

There is also an extensive list of websites where you can find more credible information about alternative therapies to traditional medical conditions.

www.webmd.com

WebMD is probably the most popular health website and includes timely and relevant news, information, educational materials, video clips, message boards, and health-care blogs, all of which are there to engage the e-patient. At WebMD, you can create a personal health record and search for a doctor or hospital, or use several worthwhile tools for information on weight and diet, a BMI calculator, advice on dental issues, skin and beauty tips, videos, a symptom checker, and more.

www.kidshealth.com

This website is sponsored and maintained by the Nemours Foundation. The Foundation is committed to supporting many health facilities and offers high-impact educational programs that affect the health of children. The site's content is divided into three separate sections—**Kids, Teens,** and **Parents**—and is written in English and Spanish. KidsHealth.com addresses a variety of subjects, from infections to mental health, from food allergies to managing asthma, from teaching kids about how the body works to helping them understand what drug abuse is all about. The information posted on the site is reviewed by physicians on a regular basis.

Finding Doctors and Hospitals

There are several websites where you can search for information about doctors and hospitals; some are more credible than others. Most of the gateway sites listed above also include search parameters for finding doctors and hospitals by geography and by subspecialty. Listed below are specific sites that are reliable, credible, and frequently updated.

www.physicianreports.com/index

At this site, individuals can search by name, state, and/or city to find a doctor, hospital, or nursing home in a particular location in the United

States. This is particularly useful for a patient who is relocating or who lives in more than one location and needs assistance in finding health-care resources.

www.ama-assn.org/aps.amahg.htm

This comprehensive web database directory of medical doctors and osteopaths practicing in the United States is sponsored by the American Medical Association. At this site, you can search by physician name or specialty. Information provided includes basic professional data such as medical school, year of graduation, board certification, telephone number, and address for both AMA members and nonmembers.

www.health.usnews.com/healthbest-hospitals/search

If you are looking for a hospital by a particular location, this website provides you with a search engine that will get you the name of the hospital in that particular geography. From that information, you can go directly to the hospital's website and evaluate whether or not it meets your criteria for size, specialized care area, etc. It is a good way to begin your quest.

Institutional Websites

One of the first places that you will turn for health information is the website of the specific hospital or medical institution that you and your doctors are affiliated with. These sites offer not only information to help you navigate the system but general information on health issues as well. Among the more comprehensive institutional sites are those sponsored by health insurers (e.g., Humana, Blue Cross, Aetna, and Kaiser Permanente).

www.mayoclinic.com

An exceptional institutional site is run by the Mayo Clinic. The content of this site is credible, reliable, and can compete with any of the health information resources available in cyberspace. In addition to the standard information about various diseases and drug listings, the site includes health tools to monitor disease; discussion options, including the ability to chat with a specialist; links to the latest health news; information and blogs; and even a first aid guide.

www.clevelandclinic.org/health

This website offers information on over nine hundred health topics, podcasts, and webcasts of health information and transcripts of web chats with physicians answering health questions. On Monday through Friday at 10:00 a.m. and 1:30 p.m., an open live chat service on this site enables you to listen to health educators on general health information and recommendations of health websites.

Professional Organizations

For patients who have a specific health problem, the best sources of information and interactive discussion groups are the sites sponsored by the associations that support those diseases. Some examples include the American Cancer Foundation, www.cancer.org..the Leukemia and Lymphoma Society, www.leukemia.org. the American Heart Association and American Stroke Association, www.americanheart.org, multiple Sclerosis, www.mspathways.com, and the Asthma and Allergies Foundation of America, www.aafa.org

Online Resources for Cancer Patients

www.cancer.gov

The National Cancer Institute (NCI) was among the first federal agencies to recognize the potential of the Internet for disseminating health-related information. The NCI site is user driven and offers cancer patients stakeholder meetings, focus groups, standard and customized online user surveys, and usability testing. The site includes information on every type of cancer and discusses new treatments and clinical trials of new drugs. As cancer patients increasingly turn to the web in large numbers seeking to be informed decision makers in their own care, NCI has responded by organizing the Cancer Net website by audience type with entry points for patients, health professionals, and researchers.

www.cancer.org

Cancer patients use Internet resources for general information about the disease as well as for pointers on how to secure a second opinion and how to interpret issues presented by health providers. For patients with rare forms of cancer, the Internet often is the only way to get support and practical advice. This site includes the hard-to-find information on the financial impact of cancer and work-related consequences. It also lists organizations offering financial assistance and provides guidelines for those of you who need to become familiar with insurance coverage, how to submit insurance claims, and help with keeping records.

www.cancercare.org

Cancercare is a nonprofit organization that provides free professional support services for individuals afflicted with cancer. At this website, there are a number of online support groups as well as education workshops where you connect in by telephone and listen to discussions on various aspects of cancer. There are also podcasts related to medical, emotional, and practical concerns of cancer patients and a comprehensive online handbook that provides financial assistance resources sorted by the type of cancer and the area where you live, within a ten mile radius of your zip code.

Online Resources for Diabetes

Diabetes is a disease in which blood glucose levels are above normal. Seven percent of the population—20.8 million people—has diabetes. About 176,500 people aged twenty years or younger have diabetes. It is a big number.

Studies have shown that online programs do work. However, there are hundreds of diabetes websites that offer suggested menus, programs, and products that are not necessarily medically approved and need to be approached with caution. There are two credible information resources on the web where you can learn everything you need to know about diabetes beyond what you learn from your own doctor.

www.cdc.gov/diabetes

This site, part of the CDC site described above, reviews symptoms, types of diabetes, risk factors, treatment options, prevention, and advice.

www.americandiabetesassociation.org

Here you'll find information on nutrition and weight loss programs, prevention, community education programs, research efforts, and more.

Web Resources for Cardiac and Lung Diseases

www.americanheart.org

This website is divided into sections for patients, caregivers, and professionals, and is full of information on how to deal with cardiac disease as well as tips on how to stay heart healthy. The Health Hub section is a patient portal where you can find tools and resources about cardiovascular disease and stroke, including a risk assessment, as well as comprehensive information to help you understand and manage your health and to determine your treatment options. Information resources include articles, podcasts, and videos. The website also has a complete description of every potential heart health condition, from arrhythmias to cholesterol.

www.nhlbi.com

At this website from the National Heart, Lung, and Blood Institute, you can find more information than you ever thought possible on heart attacks, high blood pressure, obesity, cholesterol, asthma, emphysema, lung cancer, and other issues related to heart health and lung illness. Health assessment tools are also available on this site so that you can take a more interactive role in learning about specific issues that might affect you. If you join the NHLBI Health Information Network, you will receive periodic e-mails about the latest key findings, research information, articles, and educational programs.

Web Resources for HIV

www.hivinsite.com

This is a gateway site providing information on treatment and prevention. The site is sponsored by the University of California–San Francisco School of Medicine and includes links to journal articles and academic-based information and research about

www.thebody.com

Body Health Resources Corporation launched this website for HIV-positive individuals ten years before drugs were available to prolong the lives of so many people suffering from AIDS, when there was little information out there. Over five hundred thousand visitors come to the site every month, three-quarters from the United States and the rest from around the world. A third of these visitors are people diagnosed with HIV; others are caregivers or partners of HIV-positive individuals and medical professionals. Over sixteen thousand doctors and nurses provide updates to TheBody.com. Moderated and un-moderated message boards and a variety of educational forums and materials are also available.

Weight Loss Websites

Obesity is a national health problem. In most families, there is someone who has a weight problem. Today more than one-quarter of American children are either overweight or at risk of becoming too heavy. The Internet is full of weight loss advice and services. For many adults, online diet programs are appealing. They are convenient, and you can access them any time. They offer the anonymity that many like when dealing with such a sensitive issue. Some sites include fancy tools that allow you to track your progress, which can increase your motivation to stick with a program. As with all other online health-care information, you need to be fully aware of who and what you are dealing with when reviewing weight loss programs. Many are reliable and based on good nutrition advice. Others are fad diets designed by slick salespersons who want you to purchase their products and pay high fees with few long-term results.

Three weight loss program resources that you can trust to be credible and do not try to sell you products are:

American Dietetic Association www.eatright.org

American Obesity Association www.obesity.org

Mayo Clinic www.mayoclinic.com

Web Health Resources for the Traveler

If you are about to embark on a trip outside of the United States, you know that you might encounter bacteria in the air, food, or water that can adversely impact your health. In some cases, you need vaccines when traveling to certain parts of the world. The CDC Travelers' Health site, www.cdc.gov/travel should be your first stop. Here you can find information about:

- Vaccine requirements
- Food and beverage precautions
- Swimming precautions
- Insect precautions
- Disease outbreaks (CDC Blue Sheet)

Travel Health Online, http://www.tripprep.com, is another credible website that includes updated information on vaccines, infectious diseases, health, and safety resources.

Before you leave for a long trip, you might want to locate a doctor or appropriate medical facilities in a specific geography, particularly if you have any type of chronic condition. Two organizations can offer you assistance:

International Association for Medical Assistance to Travelers www.iamat.org

International Society of Travel www.istm.org

If you plan to be way off the beaten track, you might want to check the website of the American Society of Tropical Medicine and Hygiene, www. asthm.org

Additionally you should check with your health insurance provider before you leave to determine whether or not you will be fully insured while traveling. If you are not fully insured, you might want to consider taking out travel insurance, which is available through all travel agents or at many travel sites online.

Online Drug Sites

According to Pew, nearly one-half of American adults, or about ninety-one million people, take prescription drugs on a regular basis. One in four Americans have looked online for drug information. Nevertheless the same Pew study found that only a fraction of Americans has ever bought prescription drugs online. That is slowly changing as the cost of drugs continues to rise and access to new drugs is limited and delayed by health insurers and the US Food and Drug Administration (FDA) clinical trial and approval process. Be advised that reputable sites require that prescriptions be written by a patient's health provider and adhere to regulations enforced by government agencies such as state pharmaceutical boards and the FDA. However, prescription drugs can and are being purchased at sites located in other countries where there are few if any laws or enforced policies. If you are tempted by lower drug prices and easier access on a website that may be from another country, recognize that those drugs not approved by a US regulatory agency can be compromised in dosage as well as formula and may contain contaminants, other ingredients, and even other types of drugs. You want to take proper care to insure that the drugs you are taking are in no way injurious to your health. Although no drug is 100 percent safe, best practice teaches us to order only from online pharmacies that adhere to the industry's self-regulation mechanisms, such as the Verified Internet Pharmacy Practice Site, VIPPS, run by the National Association of Boards of Pharmacy.

The FDA publishes a warning for consumers buying medical products online at www.fda.gov/oc/buyonline. The site includes a list of all drugs. If you click an individual drug, you will go to a page that will give you a complete overview of the drug and its adverse effects. For example, if you click on the over-the-counter drug naproxen, you will go to a section of the website that links you directly to a patient information sheet, a health-care provider information sheet, a prescription drug naproxen label, a paper that was issued as a public health advisory recommending limited use of Cox-2 inhibitors, and a public health advisory on nonsteroidal anti-inflammatory drug products (NSAIDS). Naproxen is one of many drugs on the market in this category.

Advice, Diagnosis, and Drugs

There are many sites on the Internet that now offer medical consults and diagnosis that are typically not covered by insurance. It is important to be vigilant about who is giving the advice, how well that individual knows you and your individual problems and health issues, and how valid the instructions are when compared to what your PCP might tell you. You should never consult a doctor who has not seen you in person at least once during the past twelve months or who does not have access to your health history, medication list, electronic health record, and other facts that are part of who you are.

Miscellaneous Useful Sites

familyhistory.hhs.gov

At this site, you can walk through the menu prompts to construct a health history of all of your family members that automatically creates a family health portrait diagram highlighting all of the specific health issues faced by various members of the family. This can be a helpful guide that you can print out and take with you to a visit with the doctor to help construct or add to your own health history and help to explain the cause of some of the issues you may be facing. It is only as useful as the information that you put into the history. You can save this information on your own computer or at Microsoft Health vault if you have an account there.

Social Networking and Health

The number of adult Internet users who have a profile on an online social network site has more than quadrupled in the past four years, from 8 percent in 2005 to 35 percent in 2008, according to the Pew Internet and American Life Project's December 2008 tracking survey. This study reinforces that Americans are aggressively pursuing health information online, particularly with the spread of wireless technology, which has unleashed a torrent of activity on e-mail lists, blogs, Facebook, Twitter, and other social networks that can be accessed not only from a desktop PC but from a wireless laptop, from a handheld PDA such as a Blackberry, and from your cell phone.

E-Patients are using social networks to ask about health and find others with the same condition at the same stage of treatment. They are comfortable talking about common illnesses as well as more complex conditions because they can get specific advice and an understanding of their options as well as reassurance that they are not the only individual suffering from this condition—something that the doctor can point out but has difficulty proving. There are issues you want to be aware of regarding social networks before you engage in interactions using these outlets:

- Do determine what your goals are if you are going to use social networking to resolve health issues or learn more about healthy problems. Stay focused on your goal and do not let fascinating, friendly people deter you from your main interest.
- Do spend some time seeking the specific people who can help you by learning the special characteristics of the search mechanisms of the social networking site and using the search to your advantage.
- Once you find a group that has relevant information for you, be sure to participate in the conversation and share information that you may have picked up with others. Doing that will ensure that the community will embrace you and help you through your issues.
- Do not get bogged down with too many social networking sites at any one time, as they all take a chunk of time and energy and can be confusing.

- Do not give away too much personal information on a social network. It can lead to misunderstanding and even trouble.
- Be astute about what good information is and what is not. Do not believe everything you are told, and try to verify any information that you given to be sure that it is reliable. For example, if you come across a new cure for acne, be sure to check out the source of the information, and before subscribing to the remedy, ask your health-care professional for an opinion.

Using social networks in health care can be daunting. The number of tools available, the sheer amount of information, the time it takes to understand and access the right groups and discussions, insuring that the information is accurate and useful—all of this is confusing and overwhelming. Furthermore most social networking sites that offer health advice are not moderated or monitored by health professionals for accuracy. The following is a breakdown of the social networks that e-Patients are typically involved with.

www.facebook.com

Currently the most popular and social networking site, Facebook's ability to connect you to a vast community of "friends" makes it easy to pose questions and find common ground on health issues that may be bothering you. You can easily create your own subgroup or join groups that have formed around health issues.

www.twitter.com

On Twitter you can engage in quick exchange of information using one simple statement of 150 characters or less. You transmit that message to fifty, five hundred, or five thousand of your colleagues, friends, or associates, provided they have a Twitter account and are following you. Your message can be a question about a health issue, a comment on a health experience, or an appeal for assistance. Twitter is a model that enables doctors to send all their patients a simple message simultaneously, such as "Flu shots are now available." You can also use Twitter to follow experts or individuals who may have similar health problems and who tweet about their experiences or offer advice. Although this may not be clinically useful, it may help you become educated. Both Twitter and Facebook help you brainstorm health problems that may be on your mind.

PatientsLikeMe

www.patientslikeme.com

PatientsLikeMe.com allows an e-patient to connect with individuals by disease or community and share data on treatments, medications, and outcomes. Active communities include ALS, multiple sclerosis, Parkinson's disease, HIIV/AIDS, many areas of mental health, and many rare diseases that do not have other websites devoted to them. New disease communities are being added constantly, and at PatientsLikeMe.com, you are invited to start a community if you have some special disease you want to talk about.

Daily Strength

www.dailystrength.org

Daily Strength is a large network of people who share advice, treatment experiences, and support. This site includes over five hundred different groups that are dealing with medical issues, mental health challenges, and life-change issues. From asthma to genetic and metabolic diseases, from mental health and addiction problems to human relations and sexuality, you can find a group to belong to. The site also includes advice and articles from medical professionals and health-care experts.

MyFamilyHealth

www.myfamilyhealth.com

At MyFamilyHealth.com, you can create a family tree, record your family health history, and assess your health risks, as well as:
- Create a medically useful record for the entire family.
- Discover and learn about health problems that run in your family, including conditions that might not otherwise be considered by your physician.

- Discover if you or your family members could benefit from specific diagnostic, genetic, or screening tests.
- Join this community and share information with others who have the same health interests as you.
- Help your physician to help you by sharing your family health history so that your physician can provide better guidance to delay, improve, or even prevent poor health that could come from genetic conditions.

ICYou

www.icyou.com

ICYou provides health videos on demand that can empower the e-patient to make informed decisions about health. From important medical breakthroughs to the latest diets, from Botox to hip surgery, plus parenting care, health-care reform, massage therapy, or education about common health practices such as hand washing, videos are available for all ages. ICYou offers thousands of videos that you can watch anytime, anywhere, as often as you like on your computer or wireless communication device at no charge. Once you register with ICYou, you are also allowed to upload your own relevant videos and share them with others in this community as well as comment on what you see. Keep in mind that although videos are an important component of acquiring health information, you need to question where these videos are coming from and who is monitoring them for health accuracy and the trustworthiness of the information.

Group Loop

www.grouploop.org

Group Loop is a social network for teens diagnosed with cancer that provides a place where teens can find same-aged individuals to talk with about their condition and treatment and open up about their emotional and social concerns while they are going though this scary, difficult time in their lives. They can also find lots of educational tips about cancer. Since so many teens have already connected through social networks such as Facebook and MySpace, Group Loop has had very wide appeal. Content includes "In the Loop," a personal profile posted each month and relayed by that individual. Another section on the website offers parents advice on dealing with their own stress and helping their teens get through this time.

Tim Berners-Lee, Director of the Worldwide Web Consortium and one of the founders of the web, described the Internet as "a universal space of information, designed to enable human communication through shared knowledge." Having the Internet available at the tips of your fingers enables you to be more informed, more in touch, and more involved with decisions that affect your life. Current technology has added a new element—collaborative virtual communication. As an e-patient, you have a responsibility to use this information access with good judgment, keeping confidential the information that you and others share through online communities and social networking and maintaining the privacy of your own health information.

Key Points

1. For every medical situation, there is a lot of good information and a lot of bad information on the web. As an e-patient, you are a seeker of the good information. Use the sites listed in this chapter as a guide because they are reliable, credible, and frequently updated to provide you with the information you need.

2. Your physician should be your primary resource for direction on how to use the Internet for medical research and what websites you should check out that have useful information on your particular health profile. Ask your physicians to supply you with a list and set up a plan to discuss questions after your web research is completed.

3. Be careful about the health products you are tempted to purchase on the Internet. Check out the contents of products to find out whether they are FDA approved and offered by a credible source.

4. Do not overlook the websites sponsored by your health insurance provider. Do not hesitate to use the customer service department for clarification regarding medications, treatment plans, questions, or observations.

5. Social networking sites offer you the opportunity for collaboration and interaction, which can help you with health-care questions and concerns. On the other hand, these sites now advertise medical products as well as other consumer goods and use tracking tools to identify what you are looking at and purchasing. Be aware that this type of monitoring could invade your personal privacy. Use these sites with caution.

6. The Internet is global, and there are many health-care sites that will try to sell you products and services that are not FDA approved and may not be in your best interest. Be sure that you are exercising good judgment. When in doubt, consult resources that you can trust.

Table 3 Best Websites

Purpose	URL	Description
Search Engines	www.google.com/tophealth/	Multilingual open content directory of web links with constantly updated content
Government Portal Site	www.medlineplus.gov	Input from over 3,000 medical Professionals; includes disease and drug database; photos; in English and Spanish
Public Health for consumers	www.cdc.gov	Travel alerts and information; public health announcements, educational materials, podcasts,
General Consumer information (government sponsored)	www.healthfinder.gov	Gateway to consumer health information from variety of government sources
General Consumer information (privately sponsored)	www.webmd.com	Timely news, information, educational tools, option to create PHR, podcasts, message boards
Family site issues	www.kidshealth.com	Special sections for kids, teens and parents with information on everything from managing asthma to food allergies. In English and Spanish
Finding a doctor or hospital	www.ama.assn.org	Database directory of doctors practicing in U.S. including basic professional information
Institutional website	www.mayoclinic.com	Information about illnesses, drug listings, discussion groups, tolls to monitor disease, chat with specialist, links to health news
Cancer	www.cancercare.org	Free professional support services; online support groups; workshops
Cardiac Issues	www.americanheart.org	Tools and resources about cardiovascular disease and stroke including a risk assessment and tools to manage heart disease
Social network	www.patientslikeme.com	An open forum where patients share health experiences, learn about the latest treatment options ; covers most disease types

Notes

1. Susannah Fox and Sydney Jones "The Social Life of Health Information," Pew Internet and American Life Project and the California Health Foundation, June 11, 2009, pp. 2–4.
2. Susannah Fox, "Health Topics," Pew Internet and American Life Project and the California Health Foundation, February 1, 2011, p. 2.
3. Ken Euteneier, Founder of the website Fibrohugs, in an interview with the author. For more information go to http://fibrohugs.com
4. *Newsweek Magazine,* April 25, 2005, p. 62.

Chapter Nine

Protecting Your Privacy

Confidentiality and Information Flow

There was a time when your personal medical information involved a conversation between you and your chosen medical provider, and no other person was involved. In modern medical practice, where numerous tests, consultations, and procedures are routine and referral to specialists by a primary care doctor is standard practice, your information is accessed by numerous faceless institutions and strangers involved directly or indirectly in the diagnosis and treatment of your medical condition or in the payment for your care. Each time you visit a doctor, therapist, hospital, or clinic, information about you is recorded and filed either on paper or, more commonly today, on a computer. Typically, this information includes a description of your symptoms, your medical history, examinations and test results, diagnoses, treatment, payment data, benefits coordination, health plan eligibility, referral certification, and authorization. Your social security number, birth date, and other relevant personal information may also be included. Third-party reimbursement, use of e-mail, e-prescribing, health information exchange, electronic medical and personal health records, and other e-health initiatives raise questions about how easily that health information can be penetrated and tampered with by unauthorized individual.

A patient at the Brigham and Women's Hospital in Boston learned that while she was an inpatient, various medical staff at the hospital had accessed her medical record more than two hundred times. Although this occurred before the passage of HIPAA and the HITECH Acts, which restrict access to your personal health information without your express consent, there are many instances when your health information is viewed by many eyes, and you may not be aware of just who is doing the viewing. For example, when you go to the emergency room of a hospital, a record is created that goes with you wherever you are transported. While the purpose is to ensure continuity of care, this record is handled by many health-care workers, including doctors-in-training, attending physicians, nurses, and technicians in all of the labs that you visit. On the general medical ward in the hospital, your record is seen by nurses, nursing assistants, residents, attending physicians, and specialists who are involved in your care. At your health plan, your health information is exposed, processed, and recorded by numerous individuals. So how do you ensure that your information is accessible only to those authorized to have access? There is no easy solution. (1)

Dave saw his primary care physician because he was having problems with his lower back, and it seemed to worsen each time he drove his car. The doctor ordered an MRI and suggested that Dave see an orthopedist. When Dave visited the specialist, he learned that two of the disks in his back were bulging and one was herniated. The doctor recommended a series of steroid injections and sent Dave to a physical therapist. Each of Dave's doctor's visits, PT sessions, and tests were billed to Dave's health plan. Three months later, Dave received a letter on health plan letterhead providing helpful suggestions on how to manage his lower back problem. Without Dave's knowledge or consent, his health plan had forwarded information about his back problem to a disease management company intended to help him. Dave was so impressed with this personalized information, he did not stop to think about whether or not he had signed permission for anyone outside the health plan view his medical information.

Although legally this kind of sharing is permitted as long as the disease management company is acting as a business associate of the health plan, had Dave's condition involved a more sensitive issue such as mental health, HIV, drugs, or alcoholism, he surely might have been upset by a third party being privy to his personal health information.

These examples raise questions about the confidentiality of your own health information that every e-patient should consider:

- How is my health information being used?
- Should I worry about the availability of my health information to so many providers and health-care workers at institutions where I receive care, individuals at my health plan, pharmacists, and others?
- Do electronic health records result in more unauthorized eyes viewing my information?
- How do I monitor what happens to my health information that is stored online (perhaps in a personal health record or in my providers' databases)?
- What can I do about maintaining the privacy of my health information?
- What recourse do I have if my privacy is violated?

Privacy is defined as "excluded or isolated from view or contact with others." Confidentiality, which should be the basis of your relationship with your doctor, is defined as "ensuring that information is accessible only to those authorized to have access." Often there are overriding legitimate reasons why health information must be shared, for instance, to avert medical error, to ensure your safety, to provide you with the necessary treatment, and to ensure that society is properly protected. There are cases where the courts have held that doctors have an obligation to pass on information to protect nonpatients, like when the doctor must warn police of a mentally unstable patient who has threatened a specific person with violence. The current health reimbursement system requires that doctors transmit medical information to payers as a condition of coverage and as a safeguard against fraud and overpayment. In most instances, your health information is sacrosanct and your privacy is maintained; however, that is not always the case.

HIPAA

There are laws regarding the privacy of your health information. In 1996 the United States Congress enacted the Health Insurance Portability and Accountability Act (HIPAA). Most consumers and even many health-care providers do not understand the fine points of HIPAA.

Title I of HIPAA protects health insurance coverage for workers and their families when they change or lose their job.

Title II of HIPAA,

This section of the HIPAA regulations, titled, *Preventing Health Care Fraud and Abuse, Administrative Simplification Medical Liability Reform*, defines numerous offenses relating to health care and sets civil and criminal penalties. It creates several programs to control fraud and abuse within the health care system. The most significant provisions of Title II are the administrative simplification rules, which establish national standards for the use and dissemination of health-care information stored on paper or in a digital format. These rules also apply to electronic health-care transactions and national identifiers for providers, health insurance plans, and employers. They address the security and privacy of health data, particularly health data that exists in digital format. As the number of consumers connecting with physicians online has increased incrementally each year since the beginning of the twenty-first century, HIPAA has gained greater importance.

The Privacy Rule

The HIPAA Privacy Rule regulates the use and disclosure of certain information held by "covered entities," generally health-care clearinghouses and employer-sponsored health plans, health insurers, and medical service providers that engage in certain transactions. It went into effect April 2003 and established regulations for the use and disclosure of Protected Health Information (PHI). PHI is any information that concerns the health status, provision of health care, or payment for health care that can be linked to you and includes any part of your medical record or payment history. It also includes a provision that outlines your right to access your medical records and control how your personal health information is used and disclosed. A key premise of the Privacy Rule is that your health information must be properly protected, while allowing the flow of health information needed to provide and promote high-quality health care to the public. Below are specifics of the Privacy Rule that are important for you to understand.

1. **Privacy practices notice:** Your providers, with certain exceptions, must ask you to read and sign a notice of privacy. This notice describes ways in which your health-care professionals may use and disclose your protected health information and includes an explanation of your right to complain to your provider and/or the Department of Health and Human Services (HHS) if you believe your privacy rights have been violated. (2)

2. **Patient access to medical records:** Upon request, you must be given control over how your personal health information is used and disclosed. You have the right to see your medical information and to copy and supplement—but not to change—your medical records. You also have the authority to refuse to have certain individuals or organizations see your records.

3. **Appropriate safeguards:** The Privacy Rule states that health-care providers, health plans, and information clearing houses that collect, share, and store health information must have appropriate technical and administrative safeguards in place to protect that information. Additionally, alternative means of communicating health information such as e-mail may be used only with appropriate safeguards.

4. **Limits on use of personal medical information:** The Privacy Rule sets limits on how health plans and providers may use your health information. There are no restrictions on your doctors, nurses, and other providers in sharing information needed to treat you. However, personal health information may not be disclosed to your employer without your written consent, nor may it be used for purposes not related to health care. Your information may be shared with a family member or other designated close friend or relative with your consent. That individual may act on your behalf to pick up prescriptions or medical supplies and provide other needed health assistance.

5. **Limits on use of health information for marketing purposes:** The Privacy Rule sets restrictions requiring you to sign a specific authorization before your providers or payers

can release your medical information to a life insurer, a bank, a marketing firm, or anyone else not directly involved in your care. While doctors and other providers and payees are permitted to communicate freely with you about treatment options and disease-management programs, marketing of your health information is not allowed.

6. **Confidential communication:** Under the Privacy Rule, you can request that your doctors, health plans, and other providers take reasonable steps to ensure that their communications with you are kept confidential. For example, you can ask a doctor to call you at a specific location rather than at home, and the doctor's office should comply with that request if it can be reasonably accommodated.

7. **Complaints:** If you have concerns about privacy, you may file a complaint using the HIPAA Health Information Privacy Complaint Form developed by the Health Privacy Project. These forms are available on the Health Privacy Project website, www. healthprivacy.org. You may also e-mail a complaint to HHS at OCRcomplaint@hhs.gov. Information on filing and updates to the Privacy Rule can be found at www.hhs.gov/ocr/discrimhowtofile. html.

The enactment of the American Recovery and Reinvestment Act of 2009 (ARRA), effective November 30, 2009, extends the complete Privacy and Security Provisions of HIPAA to business associates of covered entities, including the extension of newly updated civil and criminal penalties to business associates. Other provisions of ARRA (Section 13402-13406) tightened the privacy rule. If a business that has possession of your health information experiences a breach involving the unauthorized acquisition, access, use, or disclosure of your unsecured, protected health information that results in financial, reputational, or other potential harm to you, it must notify you or call or contact governmental authorities. This includes online companies that house your personal health record, such as WebMD, Microsoft Health Vault, and Google Health, if they are business associates. Additionally the rules regarding the marketing and communicating of products or services to you based on your health information were tightened.

The changes brought about with the passage of ARRA also require your providers and their business associates to honor a request by you to restrict disclosure of protected health information to a health plan if you have paid in full for a specific service (e.g., a second opinion) and the health plan is not involved in the reimbursement of that particular service. Further, Section 13405(d) of ARRA prohibits any direct or indirect remuneration in exchange for your protected health information without your authorization and further restricts the marketing of your health information or the marketing to you of products by vendors based on information they have obtained from your health records without your explicit permission. There are also provisions in Section 13408 of the ARRA stating that you must provide permission for transmission of your records among entities in regional health organizations, health information exchanges, or e-prescribing networks. (3)

While these federal laws and rules provide a broad umbrella under which the privacy and confidentiality of your health information is protected, state laws and common law (case law) offer even more powerful safeguards. Although there is great variance from state to state, these laws are generally more specific regarding the following:

- Written consent for the sharing of medical records, especially information that relates to sensitive medical conditions and health issues
- Issues that deal with the rights of parents and minors
- Stronger protection for specific diseases and conditions, especially HIV, mental illness, drug addiction, and alcohol addiction
- State data breach laws if your social security number of other confidential information is disclosed without authorization

State laws generally include stiffer penalties for invasions of privacy. A growing number of states have enacted identity theft laws that contain similar (but not the same) mitigation obligations as HIPAA for privacy breaches. To find out more about the laws on privacy in your state go to the state's public website and search on privacy. (4)

Privacy Violations

According to the nonprofit Privacy Rights Clearinghouse, the personal information of more than one in four Americans—eighty-five million people—was compromised between 2005 and 2006. The most publicized breach was the theft of a single Veterans' Administration laptop with the Social Security numbers and medical information of 26.5 million people that took place in the spring of 2006. An employee of the VA took the data home without authorization. Fortunately, the information was returned without damage to the security of the individuals' medical information on that laptop. However, every invasion of privacy is disturbing to the individuals who are exposed. (5)

In a survey conducted in 2005 by Princeton Survey Research Associates for the California HealthCare Foundation, respondents viewed computerization of medical information as the most serious threat to privacy. Although most of you trust your doctors to keep your information private, the survey revealed that you do not trust your health plan or government health programs to do this. Over 50 percent of respondents said that they worry about computer hackers breaking into a system that contains their medical records. That same group indicated that they trust doctors, hospitals, and other health professionals to keep personal information confidential all or most of the time. Nearly 10 percent of the respondents of this study had experienced an improper disclosure that resulted in personal embarrassment or harm. A more recent study conducted by Lake Research Partners for California Health Foundation in 2010 indicated that over 66 percent of the respondent consumers said we should not let privacy concerns stop us from learning how technology can improve health care. (6)

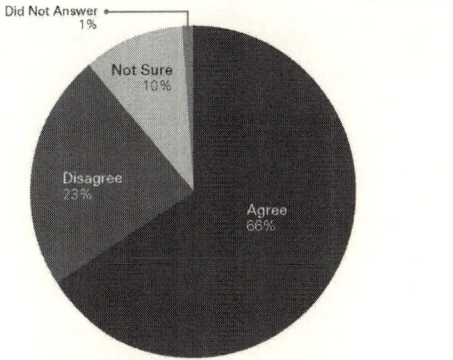

Privacy Concerns in the Use of Information Technology

Do you agree or disagree: Just like with online banking, we need to address privacy worries. But we should not let privacy concerns stop us from learning how technology can improve our health care.

BASE: ALL ADULTS (n=1,849)

- Did Not Answer 1%
- Not Sure 10%
- Disagree 23%
- Agree 66%

Source: Lake Research Partners, national health IT consumer survey, 2009–2010.

©2010 CALIFORNIA HEALTHCARE FOUNDATION. Reprinted with permission from the California Health Foundation

Health IT Consumer Survey
Privacy

Two-thirds of respondents say we should not let privacy concerns stop us from learning how technology can improve health care.

26

The proliferation of USB devices such as thumb drives, flash drives, and MP3 players creates a situation where data can be downloaded to these tiny devices and stolen with the click of a mouse. Patient files, folders, and personal information residing on the computers at HMOs, hospitals, and other health-care organizations are at risk for this type of invasion of privacy.

Even the federal government, the entity that physicians and patients assume to be the overseer and protector of the public's health information, has violated that trust. There have been several instances where attorneys for the United States Justice Department attempted to thwart privacy protections and obtain medical records. These actions were directed at the records held by Planned Parenthood clinics and were related to women who had or were planning abortions. The records sought were paper, and the Justice Department argued that the names could have been removed to protect the identification of the individuals involved. But the question remains whether or not an electronic medical record could have made it easier for the government to pry. The department justified their actions and contended that federal law does not recognize a physician-patient privilege in these instances. State courts fortunately disagreed, blocking the department's demand for access to these under the HIPAA regulations. (7)

Online Storage of Health Information

In twenty-first century health care, the increasing use of the Internet for the collection, storage, and communication of medical and other personal health records potentially enables agencies, institutions, and strangers throughout the world to view your medical records or medical information. Large databases that include these records are stored on servers connected to and accessible via the Internet. Some physicians and patients use the Internet without a secure portal to send and receive e-mail messages containing health information. Compounding the problem is the fact that many patients are required to provide personal health information to gain employment, procure insurance, obtain a credit card, or participate in today's economy. The bureaucratic institutions that control and use that information offer virtually no accountability or rationale in why or how the information will be used.

Electronic health records are generally accessed using a password protected system. Individuals with a need to see the record are typically granted access to only selective parts of the record. Audit trails closely monitor who has viewed the record. However, even with these protections, the same electronic information that sits behind firewalls and is encrypted has been subject to tampering. Then there is the issue of the privacy of e-mail communications that you elect to send, even though they include private health information. There have been many instances where patient information is shared with every good intention by providers trying to manage chronic disease issues of patients. The benefit that accrues from these activities to the patient population can outweigh any threats to privacy, but it is another slippery slope that must be approached with care. In many clinical studies, patients will provide permission for their data to be used. Generally, there is a real effort to scrub that data so that names and specific identification are not possible; however, there is always the chance that certain information could be traced back to an individual.

The Center for Medicare and Medicaid Services (CMS) has amassed databases that gather information to aid health plans, physicians, and providers in an effort to improve quality and to help Medicare beneficiaries and other consumers and health plans make informed choices. This "Quality Initiatives Research" is based primarily on information gathered directly from patients. The data is scrubbed so it is not likely that anything could be traced to specific information about individuals, but privacy issues loom whenever government collects that type of information, even if it is intended to benefit the public. (8)

The CVS Case

CVS implemented a Patient Compliance Program to provide health-care information to its pharmacy customers. Using a database prepared from customers' prescription records, a third-party company mailed letters on CVS's behalf to several of its pharmacy customers. Those customers were not previously informed of or asked to consent to this program. The mailings concerned drugs and medical conditions and took a variety of forms. Some letters provided information on the risks of certain health conditions; some letters urged customer to switch to a new or alternative prescription medication; one mailing addressed the benefits of taking and refilling prescriptions. Each letter included a box to check if the customer did not want to receive further mailings. Although the letters were written on CVS pharmacy letterhead, the mailings were financed by several drug manufacturers.

Jeffrey Kelley, who obtained his diabetes medicine at CVS, received a letter that talked about the dangers of high cholesterol, a known risk for diabetes patients. The letter was clearly marked as being sponsored by Merck and Company, Inc., a manufacturer of the anti-cholesterol prescription drug Zocor. Kelley felt that the letter invaded his privacy and, along with other individuals who had received similar letters, initiated a class action lawsuit against CVS and the pharmaceutical companies who had participated in the program. They argued that CVS and the pharmaceutical companies, for their own financial gain, improperly used confidential medical information provided to CVS by its pharmacy customers, thus violating the privacy rights of those customers.

The court held that the letter did not violate Mr. Kelley's right to privacy. In Massachusetts, an invasion of privacy requires an "unreasonable, substantial, or serious interference" with privacy. In this case, CVS did not disclose Mr. Kelley's name to Merck. They merely provided his name, date of birth, and address to the mail house. They did not know why Mr. Kelley had been selected to receive the letter and did not receive any information about his medical or pharmaceutical history. The court reasoned that there is nothing improper about a pharmacy reviewing its prescription database and providing relevant information to its customers. The fact that CVS used a third party to do this was essentially the same as hiring extra clerks to send the information directly from the pharmacy. The court also noted that Mr. Kelley "readily disclosed" his diabetes to friends and associates, which made it "even clearer that the information disclosed by CVS cannot reasonably be deemed a substantial or serious interference with his privacy." The court, however, did find that CVS engaged in an unfair and deceptive act by concealing the fact that it profited from sending the letters. (9)

The Dilemma

As a society, we cannot afford to halt progress by refusing to use electronic technology or disallowing data to be electronically stored. However, as we see from these examples, the risk that the data could be abused never quite goes away. In 1977, a group of patients and prescribing doctors brought an action challenging the constitutionality of a New York State statute that gives the state the right to maintain a database of patient names, addresses, and ages of people who use the most dangerous legitimate drugs. This data is filed with the New York State Health Department and kept for a five-year period using a system that is supposed to safeguard the security of the information, after which it is destroyed. Public disclosure of the patient's identity is prohibited, and access to the files is confined to a limited number of health department and investigatory personnel.

A case regarding the existence of this database and the privacy questions involved was heard by the United States Supreme Court (Whalen v. Roe, 429 US 589, 1977). In a unanimous decision, the court decreed that the New York program does not, on its face, pose a sufficient threat to establish a constitutional violation. The court noted that that the state's carefully designed program includes numerous words and safeguards intended to forestall the danger of indiscriminate disclosure.

We hold that neither the immediate nor the threatened impact of the patient identification requirements in the New York State Controlled Substances Act of 1972 on either the reputation or the independence of patients for whom Schedule II drugs are medically indicated is sufficient to constitute an invasion of any right or liberty protected by the Fourteenth Amendment.(10)

In a perfect world, we would have the efficiency and economies that digital technology brings to information management, collection, and storage and the privacy protections that always ensure that the data cannot be penetrated or disturbed. However, it is not such a perfect world. The digital accumulation of data has moved at a much faster pace than the ability of the same digital technology to protect that data. As these cases show, there are also many gray areas where privacy issues emerge. Therefore, the best you can do is to use all the available protections and surveillance systems available while living with the constant awareness that there are risks of your health information being disclosed or used by persons without your knowledge or consent.

What can you do to help protect your privacy? Consider the following:

- Have you provided clear instructions to your providers regarding how you want your information to be used and disseminated regarding other medical professionals they might confer with, your family and friends, your health plan, and pharmacists?
- Have you taken the proper care and considered the privacy of your health information when you put data online, particularly in respect to social networks?
- Do you assiduously avoid providing your social security number in your medical records and insist on giving out only your birth date or your provider-assigned number?
- Are you aware that if you attend a health fair or a medical screening or participate in e-mail lists, the health information you provide may not be covered by HIPAA protections or other federal and state privacy rules?
- Do you periodically ask your providers for a copy of your health record so you can review it for services provided to you and make sure they agree with your own recollection?

- Have you talked with your pharmacist about the release of your prescription information to marketing organizations and made it clear to them your desires?
- Do you keep a close check on your health insurance card, treating it like a credit card and reporting immediately if it is stolen so someone else cannot make claims against it?
- Do you carefully read the material sent to you by your health plan so that you can be sure that the benefits statement matches the services you are receiving?
- Are there opt-in and opt-out permissions that a RHIO or health information exchange allows you for the use of your data and the flow of your information among the participants in the RHIO or HIE?

Key Points

1. When you seek health care from a provider, clinic, or hospital, your health information is seen by so many health-care professionals, individuals who work for your health plan, pharmacists, therapists, and other health-care workers that there is a real danger that unauthorized individuals can access your information in spite of the laws and technology intended to prevent this from happening.
2. There are laws and regulations (HIPAA and the Privacy Rule) that establish standards for the use and dissemination of your health information, protect you, and provide you with the right to access your health information. This legislation also defines the criminal and civil penalties for abuses.
3. The American Recovery and Reinvestment Act of 2009, ARRA, tightened the HIPPA and Privacy Rule and extended coverage of these regulations to "business associates" who work with your health plan or providers to offer you additional protection.
4. State and case law further protect your health information from penetration by unauthorized individuals or groups and tend to include stricter privacy statutes than those issues by the federal government. Each state is different, so it behooves you to check out the laws specific to where you reside.

5. More than one in four Americans reports in surveys that they are concerned with privacy. It is not a trivial matter.

6. Online storage of medical and personal health records and the large databases that are amassed online as a result are inherently dangerous to the integrity of your information and the possibility that aspects of your health information could fall into the wrong hands.

Notes

1. R. Mishra, "Confidential Medical Records Are Not Always Private," *The Boston Globe*, August 1, 2000.

2. "Privacy Brief, Summary of the HIPAA Privacy Rule State Regulations," The United States Department of Health and Human Services, Office for Civil Rights, April 2003, p. 11.

3. American Recovery and Reinvestment Act of 2009 Subtitle C Section 13405(d).

4. Christopher Lee and Zachary A. Goldfarb, "Stolen VA Laptop and Hard Drive Recovered, Officials Say Data Were Not Accessed," *Washington Post,* Friday, June 30. http://www.washingtonpost.com/wpdyn/content/article/2006/06/29/AR/2006062900352.htlm

5. National Consumer Health Privacy Project, National Health IT Consumer Survey, 2005, California Health Foundation, 2009–2010 by Lake Research Partners for California Health Foundation, http://www.chef.org/topics/view.cfm/itemID=19746.

6. *Stenberg v. Carhart*, 530 US 914, 934–38 (2000); *Carhart v. Gonzales*, 331 F. Supp. 2d 805, 923–29, 1012–18(D. Neb. 2004); *National Abortion Federation v. Gonzales*, 330 F. Supp. 2d 436, 470–82 (S.D.N.Y. 2004); *Planned Parenthood Federation of America v. Gonzales*, 320 F. Supp. 2d 957, 1028–29, 1033-34 (N.D. Cal. 2004).

7. Libby Lewis, "DOJ Seeks Planned Parenthood Abortion Records," National Public Radio, http://www.npr.org.

8. www.cms.gov/qualityinitiativesgeneralinfo

9. *Weld and Kelly vs. CVS Pharmacy, Inc., et al:* Civil Action No. 98-0897-F, Superior Court Department of the Trial Court, Commonwealth of Massachusetts.

10. *Whalen v. Roe,* 429 US 589, 1977, http://biotech.law.lsu.edu/cases/reporting/whalen.html

Chapter Ten

How to Manage Your Health-Care Costs

The current health care market does not work at all like other markets. Unlike cars, computers, or retailing, for example, health-care services have not become better and cheaper over time. Instead they have become more costly and people worry about quality too. Why? Because of gross distortions in supply and demand. Consumers, the demanders, have little of the information that interests them, cannot express their feelings about the price because they rarely see the real cost of their health insurance or health-care purchases, and have an artificially constrained range of choices.

Regina, Herzlinger, Who Killed Healthcare, McGraw Hill
p.145, 2007

Ben Green received a letter from a collection agency for services rendered while his wife was in the hospital recuperating from surgery. Unknown to Ben, his employer's health insurance company refused to pay the bill for several diagnostic tests that his wife needed while hospitalized. At the beginning of the year, when Ben renewed his policy, which was offered through his employer, Ben thought he had opted for the same program he had enrolled in the previous year. However, the coverage terms had changed. Ben, who was traveling on business when the company held meetings to review policy options, had neglected to read the fine print when the policy came in the mail.

Ben's story is not unique; it is typical. Most people spend more time weighing and measuring features of a cell phone, an automobile, or a suit before making a purchase than they do considering which health insurance plan to sign up for. When they suffer a health-care crisis and find out the details of their coverage after receiving hospital bills that they cannot pay, it is too late.

By the beginning of 2000, US health spending continued to outpace inflation, rising at 7 percent annually. In 2008 health spending was over $1.9 trillion, or $5 billion a day—over 15 percent of the Gross Domestic Product. These numbers include government expenditures through Medicaid and Medicare, private health insurance, and out-of-pocket expenditures. Part of the spending problem in American medicine lies in our belief that health care is a right and not a privilege. Americans feel they should receive not only basic care but the best care that medical science can provide, no matter how they may abuse their health. Although most people contribute something to the cost of their care, they expect the rest to come from the insurer, the government, or some other source. (1)

National Health Spending
as a Share of Gross Domestic Product

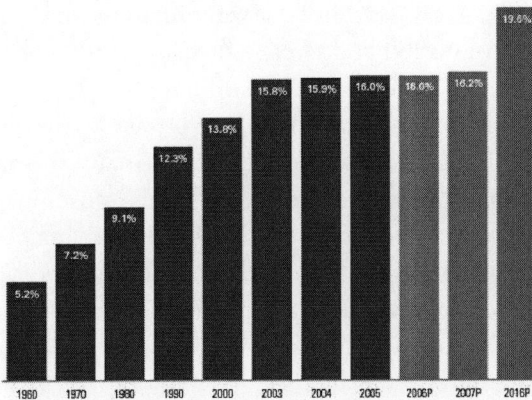

Health Care Costs 101
Spending Levels
<< PREVIOUS   NEXT >>

Health care's share of the economy continues to grow and is projected to reach 19.6 percent by 2016.

5.2% — 1960
7.2% — 1970
9.1% — 1980
12.3% — 1990
13.8% — 2000
15.8% — 2003
15.9% — 2004
16.0% — 2005
16.0% — 2006P
16.2% — 2007P
19.6% — 2016P

Note: Selected rather than continuous years of data are shown prior to 2003. Years 2006 forward are CMS projections.
Source: Centers for Medicare and Medicaid Services (CMS). Office of the Actuary.

© 2007 California HealthCare Foundations   3

In his book, *Crisis of Abundance: Rethinking How We Pay for Healthcare*, economist and author Arnold Kling writes that Americans expect "premium medicine." Kling contends that Americans routinely expect to be allowed to see medical specialists and avail themselves of advanced technology. They expect to undergo screening procedures such as MRIs, CT scans, mammograms, and colonoscopies routinely and want heroic measures during the last ninety days of life when the largest sums of health-care dollars are spent, not necessarily to anyone's benefit. Procedures such as angioplasty and heart bypass surgery are done far more frequently in the United States than in European countries, yet there is no hard data that indicates that these procedures positively affect outcomes. (2)

Poor Health Performance in the United States

A quick snapshot using data from the CDC National Center for Health Statistics:

- A study from the Commonwealth Fund comparing the quality of the US system with five other countries found that despite spending twice as much per capita, the United States ranks last or near last on basic performance measures of quality, access, efficiency, equity, and healthy lives. "The United States stands out as the only nation that does not assure access to health care through universal coverage."

- The United States ranks forty-third in lowest infant mortality rate, down from twelfth in 1960 and twenty-first in 1990. Singapore has the lowest rate, with 2.3 deaths per 1,000 live births, while the United States has a rate of 6.3 deaths per 1,000 live births. Some of the other forty-two nations that have a lower infant mortality rate than the United States include Hong Kong, Slovenia, and Cuba. The infant mortality rate is related to the underlying health of the mother, public health practices, socioeconomic conditions, and availability and use of appropriate health care for infants and pregnant women.

- For decades, the United States has been slipping in international rankings of life expectancy, as other countries improve health care, nutrition, and lifestyles. Life expectancy ranks forty-second, down from eleventh two decades earlier. Several factors have contributed to the United States falling behind other industrialized nations, including the fact that forty-five million Americans lack health insurance, while Canada and many European countries have universal health care.

- A Robert Wood Johnson Foundation study comparing the United States and ten European countries found that the United States had a much higher prevalence of nine of ten conditions, including cancer, heart disease, and stroke, in its population over age fifty. (3)
- More than 70 percent of the deaths in the United States result from behavioral and lifestyle choices such as diet, exercise, smoking, and obesity, which are primary contributors to the leading causes of death in the United States.
- More than forty million adults stated that they needed but did not receive one or more of these health services (medical care, prescription medicines, mental health care, dental care, or eyeglasses) in 2005 because they could not afford it.

Your Health-Care Choices

Mary was an accountant with one of the large national accounting firms. She loved her job and never took a sick day in the thirteen years she was with the company. She had not even bothered to find a doctor who accepted her insurance plan. At age thirty-five, Mary was diagnosed with lupus, a disease in which the immune system attacks healthy tissue. Her disease progressed rapidly, and she was unable to work and lost her job.. Several visits to her doctors, a seizure which sent her to the emergency room, high doses of expensive medications, and a requirement for CAT scans every six weeks to monitor her disease resulted in mounting bills that her insurance company began to question and eventually stopped paying. Mary was a fiercely proud woman. When the payments stopped, she stopped seeing her doctors and stopped getting tests that would monitor her disease and prevent even more insidious events. She turned to the government for assistance, but the state Medicaid bureaucracy was merely another maze to wander through. She became depressed and refused to seek further assistance. Two years after her diagnosis, Mary died of complications.

Although lupus can be fatal, most people who have it live a normal life span. The disease is usually managed with appropriate medication. However, when insurance companies refuse to pay and individuals deplete their own resources, the medications and the treatments stop, and productive citizens are not able to thrive. We know that approximately 39 percent of personal health-care expenditures are paid by private health insurance, 35 percent by the federal government, 11 percent by state and local governments, and 15 percent through out-of-pocket payments made by individuals. Of those payments, 75 percent of these health-care dollars are spent on patients with one or more chronic conditions, many of which can be prevented, including diabetes, obesity, heart disease, lung disease, high blood pressure, and cancer. We also know that throughout the first decade of the twenty-first century, health-care costs continue to skyrocket while wages remained stagnant. From 2000 to 2006, overall inflation increased 3.5 percent; wages have increased 3.8 percent; health-care premiums have increased an alarming 87 percent. Combine that with the fact that a hard-working citizen like Mary who falls ill cannot pay her medical expenses when a major medical crisis hits and you can see why health care in the United States is out of control and in a state of chaos. Approximately 50 percent of all individual bankruptcies in the United States are related to medical expenses. (4)

When you or family members are hit with a health crisis, you are likely to be outraged at the bills you are expected to pay. Fueling your anger and puzzlement is the fact that your friend in another state had the same procedure you had and paid a lot less than you are being asked to pay. The only way for you to address this confusing, dysfunctional, and unfair system is to become educated about your health plan and your options for insurance coverage. You can also choose to advocate for your right to fair and equitable health coverage. There is growing customization of health benefit plans that enables you to choose among levels of premiums, deductibles, and coinsurance as well as choices of hospitals and doctor networks. Making these choices is not easy. Although there is no one best plan—certainly not one that will cover all the costs associated with your medical care—you should try to find a plan that provides essential medical services for you and your family. Some of the questions to ask when looking for a health plan include:

- Does the plan provide the specific benefits and services you need? Are those services available quickly and efficiently?
- Can you go to the physicians and hospitals best situated for you? How easy is it to see a specialist?
- How is the plan ranked against its competitors and by its subscribers?
- Do members get the therapy treatments they need?
- Does the plan provide preventive or wellness services?
- Is the plan accredited? The National Committee for Quality Assurance (NCQA, www.ncqa.org) evaluates and rates plans on several quality measures, as does the Joint Commission on Accreditation of Healthcare Organizations (JCAHO www.jcaho.org). A visit to the websites of either of these organizations can give you rating information at no charge.

Basically there are four configurations of health plans for those who do not receive Medicare or Medicaid. The following guidelines provide you with the pros and cons of each type of health plan.

Indemnity Insurance (also called fee-for-service)

This insurance coverage pays for most of your health problems but does not typically pay for preventive care like well child visits and annual physical exams. The plan does not cover the total cost of your health care. You pay the difference with your co-pay. With an indemnity plan, you can see any doctor or go to any hospital; however, you pay a large share of the cost of the visit, even though your monthly premium is higher than any other type of health plan. Most fee-for-service plans have a "cap"—the most you will have to pay for medical bills in any one year. You reach the cap when your out-of-pocket expenses for your deductible and coinsurance total a certain amount. Over time, fee-for-service has become less desirable, since the premiums are higher than managed-care plans.

Questions to Ask About Fee-for-Service Insurance

- How much is the monthly premium, and what does that total for a year?
- What does the policy cover for specific health events? Does it include prescription drug, out-of-hospital care, rehabilitation, or home care? Does it include lab fees and emergency room visits? Do I have the option to see a specialist, and how much will that cost me out of pocket?
- Are there limits on the number of days insurance will pay for hospital or rehab services?
- Are there some medical conditions that are not be covered by the plan?
- How do you resolve treatment limit conflicts?
- Are there waiting periods involved with coverage?
- What is the deductible? Can I lower my monthly premiums by raising the deductible?
- Is there a maximum that I would pay out of pocket per year?
- Is there a lifetime maximum cap that the insurance will pay?
- How are they rated for customer service?

Managed Care, Preferred Provider Organization (PPO)

The PPO is a form of managed care closest to an indemnity plan. A PPO has arrangements with doctors, hospitals, and other providers who have agreed to accept lower fees from the insurer for their services. As a result, your cost sharing is typically lower within the network (the approved doctors in the plan) but considerably higher if you go out of the network. The PPO always includes a network of providers who have agreed to provide care to patients subject to contractually established reimbursement levels. The PPO covers many of your health-care needs for a small per-visit fee (co-payment) as long as you choose from the list of "preferred providers." You can choose to see a doctor who is not on the list, but you will pay the difference between what the provider charges and what the plan will pay, which could be significant. PPOs are the most popular form of health insurance in the United States, with over 148 million Americans participating in these arrangements.

Questions to Ask about a PPO

- What is the total annual cost of the PPO, including premiums, co-payments, deductibles, and co-insurance care for doctors outside the PPO network?
- Who are the doctors in the PPO network? Where are they located? Are they accepting new patients?
- How are referrals to specialists handled?
- What hospitals are available through the PPO?
- How is emergency care handled?
- What is their customer service like?
- Can you max out your out-of-pocket deductibles?

Health Maintenance Organization (HMO)

HMOs offer members a range of health benefits, including preventive care, for a set monthly fee. There are many types of HMOs. In some, the doctors are employees of the health plan, and you visit them at a central location. Other HMOs contract with physician groups or individual doctors who you will see in their private offices. Every HMO will give you a list of doctors from which you choose a primary care physician. That doctor coordinates your care and handles referrals when you need to see a specialist. With some HMOs, you pay nothing for an office visit, while others require a co-payment. Most HMOs cover all of your health-care needs, including checkups, immunizations, and hospitalizations, often with a co-payment. If you are forced to go "out of network" for a particular specialist that is not listed, you need to request permission, and you may have to contribute a large percentage of the charges for this service.

Questions to Ask about an HMO

- What will the HMO plan cost each year, including co-payments?
- Are there many doctors to choose from? Which doctors are accepting new patients? How hard is it to change doctors?
- How are referrals to specialists handled? What is the payment policy if a specialist is outside the HMO network?
- Is it easy to get appointments with doctors in the HMO? How far in advance must routine visits be scheduled?
- What arrangements does the HMO have for handling emergency care?
- What hospitals are in the network?
- Are there limits on services such as preventive medical tests, surgery, mental health, and home care?
- What arrangements are provided for services that are not offered by the HMO? Who covers the payments?

Point of Service (POS)

Many HMOs offer an indemnity type option known as a Point of Service Plan. The POS is basic, managed care with lower medical costs in exchange for more limited choice. When you enroll in a POS, you choose a primary care physician who must be from within the health-care network. Unlike an HMO, your POS physician may make referrals outside the network. You will pay for these services, but they are available. The advantages of a POS are that you have a much broader choice of doctors and your annual out-of-pocket costs are limited. A disadvantage is that your co-payments for non-network care are high. Overall the costs will be slightly lower than a PPO because most of your health care is controlled by your managed care insurer.

Questions to Ask about POS Health Insurance

- How many doctors are there to choose from? Where are they located?
- Are doctors in the network private or group practice?
- How are referrals to specialists handled?
- What hospitals are in the plan?
- What services are covered and are there limits to treatment?
- How much is the annual premium?
- What is the deductible for non-network care? Is there an out-of-pocket maximum?

Medicare

Medicare is the federal health insurance program for American ages sixty-five and older and for certain disabled Americans. If you are eligible for social security or railroad retirement benefits and are age sixty-five, you automatically qualify for Medicare, provided that you paid the Medicare payroll tax for at least ten years of your work life and are a citizen or permanent resident of the United States.

Medicare has three parts:

Part A helps you pay for hospital care and some other care such as home health, hospice, and skilled nursing facility care. Medicare Part A does not require you to pay a monthly fee or premium.

Part B helps pay for doctors' visits, some home health care, medical equipment, some preventive services, outpatient hospital care, physical therapy, laboratory tests, X-rays, mental health services, ambulance services and blood. With Medicare Part B, you pay a premium and have the option of choosing which coverage plan is best for you.

Part D, the prescription drug plan, subsidizes the costs of prescription drugs for Medicare beneficiaries. Under the Medicare Modernization Act, as of January 1, 2006, insurance companies and other private companies are mandated to work with Medicare to offer Part D drug plans and determine discounts on drug prices. These drug plans vary in terms of what prescription drugs are covered, how much you have to pay, and which pharmacies you are allowed to use. People with an income at or below a set amount and with limited resources will qualify for extra help under Medicare Part D. This help is intended to assist you with a drug's monthly premium and with costs you would normally have to pay for prescriptions.

Medicare includes two approaches that you may choose from:

1. **The Original Medicare Plan** is a traditional fee-for-service plan where you can choose any doctor or hospital you want and Medicare will pay a share of the costs while you pay the rest.

2. **Medicare Managed Care Plans** offered by private insurance companies pay for the same services as the Original Medicare Plan as well as for additional health care services where you pay a co-payment every time you visit the doctor, hospital, or use other health-care services. These plans are available in most but not all parts of the country.

In other words, Medicare is a subsidized service, not a free service. How much you pay depends on which plan you choose, how often you go to the doctor or hospital, whether you have other health insurance, and whether you qualify for help through other state and publicly supported health programs.

Medigap

You may want to consider purchasing a private insurance policy called medigap to pay medical bills that Medicare does not cover. Medigap policies are sold by private insurance companies to fill the "gaps" in original Medicare plan coverage, and their terms are regulated by federal and state statutes. There are twelve different standardized medigap policies (medigap plans A through L), and their costs vary.

The best information on Medicare is found in the Medicare Handbook, which explains how the Medicare program works and what your benefits are. To order a free copy, write to the Health Care Financing Administration, Publications N1-26-27, 7500 Security Blvd, Baltimore MD 21244-1850. Or call 1-800-MEDICARE, the twenty-four-hour customer service line. You can also find answers to your questions about Medicare at www.medicare.gov.

Consumer Directed Health Plans (CDHP)

The Bordens are a middle-class American family with two young children, a modest home with a mortgage, a dog, two cars, and a couple of credit cards that always seem to have a monthly balance larger than the Borden's budget. Although both parents work and have received cost of living wage increases over the past several years, there never seems to be enough money to make ends meet. An analysis of their budget reveals that higher payroll deductions from Dad's paycheck for health care, which covers the entire family, and higher out-of-pocket expenses for medical needs during those same several years has exceeded their cost of living raises.

This same story repeats itself in family after family across the country. Two hard-working citizens making a genuine contribution to society are being financially buried, many even becoming bankrupt, due to the burden of critical health-care expenses. Receiving state-of-the-art of health care is unachievable for the average American family today. For years, health-care spending has been in the purview of insurers, the government, or your employers. They determine what medical expenses and tests will be covered and what will not. If you opt for a service not covered, you pay for it, in spite of the high premiums you pay each month.

This burden of deciding how to spend health-care dollars is shifting from government agencies, your employer, and insurers to you. A growing movement in the health-care system is putting more responsibility for the cost of health insurance benefits and the purchase of health services on you through consumer directed health plans (CDHPs). CDHPs were devised by health policymakers to reduce health-care costs while offering optimal health-care coverage that meet your needs. The CDHP model is based on your having all the necessary information to make informed decisions. Access to digital communications that empower you and support your ability to make decisions about how to spend your health dollars are an underlying component of CDHP. Additionally, with your own money at stake, a more competitive marketplace emerges, where insurers are forced to provide more cost-effective programs, and providers must become more efficient and cognizant about the cost of the care they deliver. An argument in favor of CDHPs is that they lower health-care costs by making you a better shopper for health-care services. The basic arrangement for CDHPs includes high-deductible insurance plans combined with a savings account option that CDHP enrollees can use to pay for routine or extraordinary health expenses with tax-deferred funds. There are three configurations:

- **Health Savings Accounts (HSA)**—These are created by individuals who are covered by a qualified health plan that has a high deductible to assist them in paying out-of-pocket health expenses. Both employees and employers can contribute to an HSA up to an annual limit set by a statutory cap. Employee contributions to an HSA are made on a pre-income tax basis, and some employers arrange for contributions through payroll deduction. The HSA is owned by the individual, who retains the funds if he/she were to leave the job

- **Health Reimbursement Accounts (HRA)**—HRAs are medical care reimbursement plans established by employers and used by employees to pay for health care. Employers typically commit to a specific amount of money available in the HRA for an individual to pay premiums and other medical expenses. Unspent funds in an HRA are usually carried over to the next year. Employees do not take their HRA balance with them if they leave the job.

- **Flexible Spending Account (FSA)**—The flexible spending arrangement allows an employee to set aside a portion of his or her earnings to pay for qualified expenses, most commonly for medical expenses but also for dependent care or other expenses. Money deducted from an employee's pay and put into an FSA is not subject to payroll taxes, resulting in a substantial income tax savings. Paper forms or an FSA debit card, also known as a flexcard, may be used to access account funds. The FSA is similar to both HSAs and HRAs in that these funds are set aside to pay health-care expenditures. However, while HSAs and HRAs are almost exclusively components of a consumer-driven health-care plan, medical FSAs are commonly offered with more traditional health plans.

Where Do You Get Health Insurance?

In making an employment decision, health benefits have become one of the most important factors, second only to wages. Employers, being well aware of this, are straining to stay solvent and offer the benefits their employees need. It is not easy. Starbucks spent more on employee health insurance in the year 2005 than on raw materials to brew its coffee. Starbucks provides health-care coverage to all employees who work at least twenty hours a week, which management feels is key factor in the company's low employee turnover and high productivity.(6)

Jeanie is a financial analyst who has been working for one of the large banking institutions for ten years. Her husband is an independent consultant and works for himself. They have three children. The family's health coverage is provided through Jeanie's employer. Jeanie has often thought about starting her own business, but the bank provides comprehensive health insurance. As an entrepreneur, she would have to find coverage elsewhere. Since her daughter has asthma and her son requires frequent checkups for junior rheumatoid arthritis, Jeanie is unhappily locked into her job because she cannot risk the loss of this health coverage for herself and her family.

Most Americans get health insurance through their employer, a family member, an association, or other group. Employers negotiate group policies that are typically considerably less expensive than individual plans. Some employers offer only one health insurance option, but most give you a choice of plans (i.e., fee-for-service plan, HMO, POS, or PPO). As the cost of health insurance has increased, the number of choices employers offer has decreased, and the health-care burden grows more cumbersome for everyone. Usually when you choose a health plan, you must keep it for the year. During the open enrollment period at the end of the year, you can choose another option if it is offered.

If you or your family member leaves the job that provides your health insurance, you will lose your employer-supported group coverage. A federal law, the Consolidated Omnibus Budget Reconciliation Act of 1985 (COBRA), makes it possible for most people to continue their group health coverage for a period of eighteen months after leaving a job. You pay the full premium at the group rate.

Not all employers offer health insurance. You can find group insurance through membership in unions, professional associations, and other organizations. Individual insurance is available under fee-for-service, HMO, and PPO arrangements, but the coverage and the costs vary and are often prohibitive.

Before buying any health insurance policy, you need to be sure that you know what it will pay for and what it will *not* pay for. The following tips should help you shop for individual insurance:

1. Shop carefully; policies differ widely in coverage and cost.
2. Make sure the policy protects you from large medical costs.
3. Read and understand the policy, including the fine print. You do not want surprises when you are sick or in the hospital.
4. Check to see when the policy will begin paying and what is covered or excluded.
5. Make sure there is a "free look" clause—a period to look over the policy after you receive it to decide whether or not it is right for you.
6. Beware of single-disease insurance policies that offer protection only for one disease, such as cancer. A basic policy should cover everything, so you do not need these additional protections, which can be expensive.
7. Determine what type of insurance works best for your personal situation—basic coverage or more comprehensive coverage? Do you need access to specific doctors at specific locations? Can you afford higher out-of-pocket payments, or do you need to be with a plan that requires very little out-of-pocket expense? (17)

The Patient Protection and Affordable Care Act (PPACA)

When Dan was laid off from his engineering job, he lost not only his work, his income, and his feeling of self worth, but his health insurance as well. COBRA payments were out of the question, as Dan did not have the resources to keep up with the premiums. Diagnosed with depression six months after the layoff and unable to find other work, Dan also lost his condo, his car, and his credit cards, and he ended up homeless. Having had asthma all of his life, Dan developed breathing problems and contracted pneumonia. He landed in the emergency room of a large urban public hospital and was admitted. Dan became one of nearly fifty million uninsured American individuals who should have some recourse for finding health care before an illness or a chronic condition precipitates into a major crisis that risks his life and sends health-care costs for everyone spiraling upward. In a bad economy, this situation could happen to anyone.

PPACA, signed into law on March 23, 2010, has been the subject of much heated discussion, political posturing, and debate. It is clear that US health-care expenditures that are at 16 percent of GDP are not buying us the kind of healthy life that is enjoyed in other countries. The reform elements in the PPACA attempt to address some of these deficiencies and make things better. Here are a few highlights of the bill that you need to understand:

1. Beginning in 2011, insurance companies are required to spend at least 80 percent of the premium dollars they collect on direct medical care and quality improvement activities. Furthermore, they must publicly report how they spend those dollars. This should help reduce health disparities, bring down health-care costs, increase investment in prevention and wellness, and give you and your family more control over your care.

2. Starting with plan years beginning on or after September 23, 2010, the law requires health plans and health insurance policies to cover certain recommended preventive services at no charge to patients in an effort to encourage you to live a healthier life. This includes:

   a. Medicare patients will be eligible for an annual wellness exam and certain preventive services with no cost-sharing.

   b. States and local communities will be given new resources to address chronic diseases, obesity, smoking, and drug use.

   c. Additional provisions enable consumers who have joined new health plans to receive cost-free preventive services like regular check-ups, cancer screenings, and immunizations at no additional cost; the choice of a primary care doctor, ob/

gyn, and pediatrician of your choice; and the ability to use the nearest emergency room without penalty

3. The act has a provision that enables you to keep young adults on a parent's plan until age twenty-six.

4. It includes a mandate that insurers will no longer be able to deny coverage to children with preexisting conditions, place lifetime limits on benefits, cancel a policy retroactively without proving fraud, and deny claims without the chance for appeal.

5. The law forbids insurers from refusing to cover you on the basis of preexisting conditions and prevents your health plan from assessing you with a higher co-payment or co-insurance for out-of-network emergency room services.

6. The law bans insurance discrimination so people who have been sick can't be excluded from coverage or charged higher premiums, including women who no longer have to pay higher premiums because of gender.

7. The Affordable Care Act mandates a new health insurance marketplace by 2014 consisting of health insurance exchanges that offer one-stop shopping so individuals can compare prices, benefits, and health plan performance on easy-to-use websites. The exchanges will guarantee that all people have a choice for quality and affordable health insurance even if a job loss, job switch, move, or illness occurs. The new law also provides tax credits to help Americans pay for insurance.

8. The law expands initiatives to increase racial and ethnic diversity in the health care professions. It strengthens cultural competency training for all health-care providers and requires health plans to use language services and community outreach in underserved communities.

9. The act expands the health-care workforce and increases funding for community health centers, including health teams that can manage chronic diseases and comprehensive health services for everyone, no matter how much they are able to pay.

10 The PPACA law provides new funds for home visits for expectant mothers and newborns in an effort to reduce infant mortality and post-birth complications.

11. New rules included in the Health Reform Act will simplify paperwork for physicians and lessen their administrative hassle.

This, along with investments in electronic health records, will help doctors and hospitals focus more on patient care and less on paperwork.

12. Investments in new models of patient-centered, coordinated care, including investments in medical homes and other advanced care coordination and disease management tools, will give you more control over how your care is delivered and enable your providers to be rewarded with bonuses when they meet certain criteria.

13. PPACA supports the training and development of more than sixteen thousand new primary care providers over the next five years and establishes new nurse-managed health clinics to train nurse practitioners to work in underserved communities. It also provides the structure for The National Health Service Corps, a program that repays loans and gives scholarships to primary care providers who work in areas of the country with too few health professionals.

14. Starting with policies issued or renewed on or after September 23, 2010, insurance companies will be prohibited from dropping patients from coverage when they get sick because of an unintentional mistake on a form. By 2014, annual limits are phased out that adversely affect the sickest patients with the highest costs.

15. Provisions that went into effect on September 23, 2010, address the Medicare drug coverage gap, also called the "donut hole." This means that after you and your plan have spent a certain amount of money for covered drugs, you have to pay all costs out-of-pocket for your drugs (up to a limit). Starting in 2011, if you have high prescription drug costs that put you in the donut hole, you'll get a 50 percent discount on covered brand-name drugs while you're in the donut hole. Between 2010 and 2020, you'll get continuous Medicare coverage for your prescription drugs.

16. The new law extends the life of the Medicare Trust fund at least twelve years and takes other actions to secure the program.

17. The legislation does not make any changes in COBRA. Coupled with that, the Early Retiree Reinsurance Program (ERRP) provides much-needed financial relief to businesses, schools, and other educational institutions, unions, state and local governments, and

nonprofits in order to help retirees and their families continue to have quality, affordable health coverage.

At the website www.healthcare.gov, you will find answers to additional questions you may have. This website has tools to help you assess quality of health-care delivery organizations and provides links to www.healthfinder. gov where there is extensive information on prevention and wellness, including an encyclopedia with over 1,600 health topics, resources to help you find doctors and hospitals, the latest health news from research studies, and a quick guide to healthy living, including activity and menu planners.

Key Points

1. US health-care spending is nearly 16 percent of the gross domestic product, twice as much as most other countries, with not very much to show for these expenditures when evaluating our mortality rates and other basic quality performance measures.
2. Our personal health-care costs continue to rise at an alarming rate, with higher premiums and higher out-of-pocket expenses, while our wages have dropped significantly relative to inflation. Therefore, even those of us who have health insurance are grossly underinsured in the event of a major catastrophic medical event.
3. To enrage us even more, health-care costs are uneven, with the cost of a procedure in one area of the country or even in one institution within a specific geography vastly different than the cost of the same procedure elsewhere.
4. Individuals have to become significantly better informed about the specifics of their health insurance policies and their options when choosing a health plan.
5. There are good and bad elements in each of the health plans currently available that include: indemnity insurance, managed care with a preferred provider organization, HMOs, and point-of-service plans.
6. For those over the age of sixty-five who are eligible for Medicare, the issues are complex. It is best to seek assistance either online

at www.medicare.gov, or by ordering a free copy of the Medicare Handbook.

7. Consumer Directed Health Plans enable individuals who get their health insurance through their employers to set aside some health-care dollars in an HAS, an HRA, or a flexible spending account. This places an added burden on you to become an educated consumer but helps pay those unexpected medical costs that inevitably crop up.

8. The Patient Protection and Affordable Care Act is complex and detailed. There are many elements in the act that will improve your access to care over time that you need to be aware of. You will find that information at www.healthcare.gov.

Notes

1. "Snapshot Health Care Costs 101", California Health Foundation, 2007.
2. Arnold Kling, "The Rise of Premium Medicine," *Crisis of Abundance: Rethinking How We Pay for Health Care,* Cato Institute, Washington D.C., 2006.
3. Elizabeth Doctor and Robert Berenson, *"How Does the Quality of U.S. Healthcare Compare Internationally?"* Robert Wood Johnson Foundation, Urban Institute, 2009.
4. David Himmelstein, Elizabeth Warren, et al., "Market Watch: Illness and Injury as Contributors to Bankruptcy," *Health Affairs Journal,* February 2005, doi:10.1377 hlthaff.w5.63.
5. "Faces in the News," *Forbes Magazine*, Sept 15, 2005.

Chapter Eleven

Health Care 2050: Your Medical Future and You

At its very core, our work today is about improving lives and ensuring peace of mind. It's about getting the right care to the right person at the right time—each and every time . . . Today, one out of five Medicare patients who leaves a hospital is back within thirty days. Often, this is because patients don't get the right follow-up care: they didn't understand their doctor's directions, they didn't eat the right diet or take the right medicines, or get the right wound care.

Katherine Sibelius Secretary, Department of Health and Human Services, National Summit on Health Care Quality and Value, Washington, D.C., October 4, 2010.

Technology to the Rescue

Baby James is born on February 12, 2050, at 3:00 a.m. Minutes after his birth, a microchip the size of a grain of rice is embedded in his arm. It is coded with an assigned number that will belong to James for the rest of his life, no matter where in the world he may go, and points to a secure website that was created within hours of James's birth. Stored at this site are all of the tests administered to James in his first few days of life, including the PKU, the APGA, James's blood type and DNA, genetic markers, analysis of James's stem cells and skin tissue, results from a hearing test, a thumb print, and a scan of his retina, as well as his birth certificate and other important information. James (or his family until he becomes of age) will own and control access to this record. It will be available on a need-to-know basis to all his health-care providers, with consent. This immediate access to James's information eliminates the need for duplicate tests or interventions. It provides the right information for James, no matter where or when he needs care.

Imagine the Possibilities

Imagine a world where every person has a microchip that lasts indefinitely and transmits a unique fifteen-digit number that can be read by a handheld scanner that points to your digital health record every time you see a health-care provider or go to the emergency department. The doctors who take care of you can add comments and updates to the record to keep it current. You can also enter data in your record.

Imagine a time when electronic devices linked to computers and communications networks allow your implants and medical conditions to be monitored remotely at any time.

Imagine having an operation done by a robotic arm equipped with laser beams that repair, extract, and replace tissue and organs. The procedure is not invasive and enables you to go home from the most intricate surgery hours later. Your doctor is right there overseeing the operation, available to answer your questions and jump in if there is an emergency.

Imagine knowing years before it might happen about a disease you are carrying that is detected by noninvasive brain scans that can also look at the impact of various drugs or chemical imbalances on your body, enabling your doctors to engage in preventive measure that could markedly increase your life span and quality of life.

Imagine having the ability to protect yourself against neurological conditions such as Alzheimer's disease, ALS, Parkinson's disease, or the ravages of cancer by understanding the genetic markers you are born with.

Imagine that when you brush your teeth, your toothbrush examines your gums and takes your blood pressure, blood sugar, and oxygen levels.

Imagine that when you step out of bed, your carpet measures your weight.

Imagine that when you go to the bathroom, your toilet diagnoses your current body chemistry and detects irregularities in your waste.

Imagine that all of this information is collected and transmitted through your smartphone or computer to a remote location where nurses are monitoring you and addressing any irregularities that they detect before they result in a visit to the doctor or the emergency department.

All of these changes and more will be standard in the health care you experience in the second half of this century. They will be made possible with sophisticated diagnostic digital tools available to you and to your physicians. In the next several years, more technology, greater insight into the mechanisms of the human body, better education, and incentives that empower you as a patient will result in the adoption of these and as-yet-unimagined discoveries. Communication, convergence, and implementation of standards and protocols will make interconnection as transparent as telephone or e-mail communications are today. This easy transfer of information will result in a continuous patient-centered care model that will become the norm.

Devices and Enablers

There are a number of devices that were developed in the twentieth century and the first decade of the twenty-first century that make Health Care 2050 and beyond possible.

Personal Digital Assistants

PDAs started out as mobile phones with calendars and address books; e-mail, Internet access, cameras, and GPS devices that can actually pinpoint a patient's exact location were added. These personal digital assistants evolved into smartphones and tablet computers, for which there are several thousand applications for health care, including apps that can transmit a patient's blood pressure, heart rate, and other vital signs, as well as a graphic image of an individual or a specific part of the body that requires examination. These same smartphones and tablets provide physicians with access to drug information and intelligent decision support tools for immediate accurate diagnostic assistance. The potential is limitless as smartphones become a diagnostic and research device that promises enormous benefits to e-Patients and their physicians. (See Table 4, Best Free Smartphone Apps.)

Radio Frequency Identification (RFID)

RFID is a technology where tiny transmitters embedded in a tag or bracelet send out an encoded stream of bits to alert a reader. During the first decade of the century, RFID technology was used to match an identifier on a patient with an identifier on a pill container or other medication container to check that the right patient is given the right drug at the right dosage. RFID has also been used to track materials, medications, and patients in the hospital to reduce medical error and promote patient safety. This includes specimen collection, blood and medication administration, nursing workflow and tracking processes, patient movement, and tracking medical equipment throughout the hospital. RFID makes the environment safer for the e-patient and more efficient for medical institutions and the physicians to treat patients.

Robots

Robots with built-in microprocessors and sensors are capable of performing a variety of complex human tasks on command by remote control. Health-care robots are equipped with a set of medical sensors enabling them to multitask. They can measure blood pressure, heart rate, heartbeat irregularities, and body temperature. Robots help in the care of the elderly or chronically ill patients in addressing cognitive decline by reminding patients to drink, to take medicine, or to remember an appointment. They are also used for collecting data, monitoring for emergencies such as heart failure, and assisting people with domestic tasks.

By the beginning of this century, robots capable of performing complex assignments were developed to assist human surgeons in performing minimally invasive surgery. Since their precision is extremely accurate, they reduce the number of people needed in the operating room and enhance surgical performance with their superior dexterity. By the second half of the century, robotic telepresence, which allows physicians to conduct remote patient rounds, consult with staff, and access patient data via two-way real-time streaming video, wireless protocols, and the Internet, will be commonplace. Even today in some VA hospitals, a six-foot tall robot equipped with a fifteen-inch flat screen, two high-resolution cameras, and a microphone engages in two-way video conferencing as it makes rounds and sees patients. A live conversation and visit between patient and the doctor, who remotely controls the robot through an Internet connection, takes place. The physician appears on the screen and carries on a conversation with the patient as easily as if he or she were physically present. The doctor remotely drives the robot through the hospital to each patient's room to check vital signs, inspect incisions, and discuss treatment options in real time. In the future, specialists who may be hundreds of miles away will also use robots to virtually consult with patients. There will be robots that help in the emergency room and other robots that will monitor patients in the intensive care unit working with a physician who is sitting in a remote location. This takes the eICU to another level.

Telemedicine

Telemedicine, which has been limited by legislation and funding, will be much more widespread by 2050. In large urban centers and in remote geographies, telemedicine that enables remote diagnostic patient/physician visits, treatment of trauma cases right at the site of the emergency, and home monitoring services for elderly and home-bound patients who cannot get to the doctor or the hospital for care will become available to everyone because it is an efficient and economic way to deliver health care.

Personalized Medicine

On October 27, 2005, the International HapMap consortium published a comprehensive catalog of more than one million human genetic variations. This HapMap database allows researchers to compare the genetic sequences of different individuals. What began as research collaboration among scientists from several countries across the world has changed the way medical professionals understand the origins of illnesses and how to prevent, diagnose, and treat those illnesses.

Personalized medicine is founded on the principle of providing customized health care to individual patients based on their genetic makeup. Your genes define your risk factors for many common diseases and guide your physicians in providing you with optimal preventative and therapeutic care. Up to now, personalized medicine has been limited to consideration of your family history, social circumstances, environment, and behaviors in tailoring your individual care. In the future, your doctors will be able to test your DNA and check for variations that not only identify potential disease, but also enable them to draw conclusions regarding adverse reactions to a broad range of drugs and treatments.

DNA sequencing of individuals is now possible, but there are cost and philosophical barriers to its wide acceptance. By 2050, DNA sequencing will result in customized patient care for everyone based on their genetic makeup. E-Patients, unless they opt out, will know their risks and will be able to make appropriate lifestyle changes and engage in more aggressive disease surveillance and preventive medical treatments. By 2050, genetic variants that contribute to longevity or provide information related to resistance to disease will provide pathways for new therapies with widespread benefits. This personalized, information-based health care, which rests on scientific information and not conjecture, will transform medicine, enabling your physician to know what works, why it works, and who it works for.

The Practice of Medicine in 2050 and Beyond

The cornerstone of health-care practice in 2050 will be that the patient occupies center stage. Interactions between patients and provider will take place whenever and wherever feasible, via face-to-face visits in the doctor's office, at a house call, on a web portal, on a smartphone, in a quick response clinic, or, as a last resort, in the hospital emergency department. All fundamental health-care services will be provided to individuals by a health-care gatekeeper, who will be responsible for coordinating care, controlling costs, and communicating results. Advances in telecommunications, medical imaging, massive intelligent databases, satellite technology, and other information systems will allow physicians to communicate far more easily and quickly, and will enable patients to educate and empower themselves to take responsibility for their health.

183

Patients will be served in a number of ways. Those who live in urban and suburban centers and who are too elderly or infirm to leave their place of residence will be visited at least quarterly by a core of physicians who, along with their nurses and nurse practitioners, will make house calls. These same patients will be monitored daily at the telemedicine centers. Face time with your physicians will be supplemented with web visits. Portable computing technology, tablets, smartphones, access to patient portals, and the assistance of robots will prevent illness from escalating out of control. For mobile patients, there will be a number of ways to access health care. Retail clinics, which became a factor early in the century, will spread across the country and will be available to everyone for routine problems. There will be less fragmentation in health-care delivery as e-Patients find their own medical home, whether with a group medical practice endorsed by their insurer or through a concierge practice that they opt to engage with flexible spending accounts that they have amassed in conjunction with their employment benefits package. For the poor and uninsured, community health centers will offer comprehensive health-care services and serve as their medical home.

The task of managing the resources of healing is one of the most complex chores individuals must face. By the second half of the century, a realignment of provider networks into patient-centered care management groups will offer you continuous care whenever and wherever you need it. Wireless networks will release you from having to communicate from a specific location. You can access health-care assistance whether you are in the car, at the office, at the beach, watching a movie, or working out in the gym. You can proactively send images, video, and audio descriptions to your health providers remotely. Feedback is fast and efficient. Routine tests and examinations that used to require an in-office visit are done remotely via connected EKGs, EEGs, and portable telehealth units that include tactile devices in the form of hats, gloves, floor mats, bracelets, and toothbrushes that communicate via your smartphone or tablet.

The overall cost of health care will continue to rise due to an aging world population. During the first half of the century, the global population of individuals age sixty or over is projected to expand by more than a factor of three. By 2050, one in every three persons living in the more developed regions of the world is likely to be sixty or older, and about one in every four is projected to be sixty-five or older. (1)

During the last sixty to ninety days of life, there is a disproportionate amount of money spent on an individual's health care, which impacts resources available throughout the system. By 2050, there will be different payment processes and formulas than currently exist. A coalition of government, private organizations, employers, hospitals, physicians, payers, and foundations will oversee how we pay for care, who pays what, and how to overcome the inequities in the system. A series of tax incentives and legislated regulations will mandate that employers large and small provide all employees with basic health care during their work tenure and for several months after they cease to work as an employee unless they opt out. Small companies that cannot afford this coverage will be assisted through federal programs and quasi-public agencies set up for this purpose. Extraordinary health expenses will come out of an individual's health account that you set up either with matching grants from your employers or with personal funds. Individuals who cannot afford health accounts, who are unemployed, disabled or otherwise unable to work, will be supported by public funds. However, they are the only individuals who will be supported by public funds, as Medicare and Medicaid will have been cut way back.

In 2050, you will be offered incentives and will be provided with the education that keeps you on track regarding health issues. In addition to the fact that you will have mobile devices to stay in close communication with your e-health professionals, you will be more thoroughly briefed in how diet, blood pressure, blood sugar, cholesterol, and other critical markers that impact your health should be kept in check. Adherence to medication, a weight plan and an exercise program, and control of tobacco and alcohol intake will be rewarded with lower rates for your health-care coverage, similar to the penalty/reward system used today by auto insurers. This is part of the high value that is placed on healthy living. Additionally, a system of online social health networks will support you through extraordinary health events.

Privacy issues still loom large in health care in 2050. The more digital data we have, the more there is to be penetrated, and although the points of entry are more tightly controlled with advanced encryption technology and scanning capabilities (retinal scanning of individuals before accessing a record), there is always an underlying threat. Human nature being what it is, patients in 2050 will have reason to fear that with sophisticated digital records, savvy individuals or companies who desire to access those records for profit or illicit purposes can and will do so.

By 2050 every medical school will have incorporated health information technology into their curriculum so that graduating physicians have undergone training in the benefits and the logistics of electronic health records, telemedicine, Internet resources, CPOE, privacy issues, and business questions related to HIT. This change in training produces physicians who are more entrepreneurial and open to a constantly changing health-care landscape, promulgating more rapid adoption of new technology, better communication with patients, and more evenly divided resources.

Key Points

1. The availability of information technology that fosters the potential for twenty-four-seven communication between e-health professionals and e-Patients forms the essence of their relationship in Health Care 2050. Patients are the cornerstone and are served in many ways, from home monitoring to retail clinics to web visits to traditional care in the doctor's office or at the hospital. With their mobile devices, they are an integral part of the health-care team.
2. A microchip embedded in every individual in 2050, which points to a personal health record residing on a secure site on the Internet, resolves the issue of who owns your digital health record and how it is accessed by the your providers.
3. Patients in 2050 are educated, motivated, and incentivized to pay attention to their health and work toward a healthy lifestyle, thus curbing some of the demand for health-care services.
4. Many devices and enablers, including smartphones, tablet computers, RFID, robots, extensive telemedicine networks, and

decision support systems, all based on sophisticated wireless technology, foster better, safer medicine for everyone.

5. Basic health coverage is the norm in 2050. Those who are employed receive their care in their benefit package from their employers. They have to save and pay for their extraordinary health expenses, however, which are not as readily available through their health coverage as they had been. Those who are not employed, such as seniors, children, and disabled individuals, have access to health-care coverage through a collaborative of private and public funds.

6. Physicians are taught in medical school and continuing education programs about the logistics and value of information technology, and it becomes part of their everyday professional life.

7. Personalized medicine, based on our understanding of the human genome, has changed medicine by 2050, including more effective ways to predict individual susceptibility to disease, more useful and person-specific tools for preventing disease, greater ability to detect the onset of disease based on markers, and preempting the progression and severity of disease.

Table 4

Major Trends in Healthcare

Trend	Impact	Challenges
Electronic Health Records	Instant access to information; decision support tools	Privacy of health information
Personal Health Records	Empowered patient	Keeping the record up to date
Smartphones	Instant access to health information	Filtering good apps from bad
Email	24/7 asynchronous communication	Focusing on the issue and keeping the email concise
e-Visit	Saves money and time by eliminating unnecessary office visit	Insuring the interaction is meaningful; e-Visiting only with physician you know
e-prescribing	Elimination of medication error, speed in obtaining medication	Medication adherence if reasons for drug are not properly explained
Retail Clinics	Fast and economical way to address minor ailments	Integration with primary care physician
Nurse Practitioners and Physician assistants providing primary care	Addresses shortage of PCPs and enables more people to access basic medical care	Insuring best practices; determining when to refer to MDs
Telemonitoring	Keeps people in their home	Reimbursement, dependence on patient understanding and cooperation
Payers influence in care decisions	Healthcare driven by finances and not specific medical issues	Maintaining integrity of care
Internet	Information access, collaboration, research, communities	Information overload and quality issues

Notes

1. *World Population Aging: 1950–2050,* US Department of Economics and Social Affairs, Population Division, for the 2002 world Assembly on Aging, Chapter IV, p. 23.

GLOSSARY OF TERMS

adherence: Patients' following a prescribed treatment ordered by a physician, including the taking of medications at the times and dosages prescribed.

Agency for Healthcare Research and Quality (AHRQ): Part of the US Department of Health and Human Services. AHRQ supports research to improve the outcomes and quality of health care, reduce costs, address patient safety and medical errors, and broaden access to effective services.

The American Recovery and Reinvestment Act of 2009 (ARRA): Includes the Stimulus Act with a provision that provides financial incentives for physicians to implement electronic health records.

Centers for Disease Control and Prevention (CDC): A federal agency within the Department of Health and Human Services that serves to enhance and promote the health and quality of life of US citizens by preventing and controlling disease, injury, and disability. Working with states and other partners, CDC's system of health surveillance monitors and prevents disease outbreaks, including bioterrorism. CDC also implements disease prevention strategies, maintains national health statistics, and provides for immunization services, workplace safety, and environmental disease prevention. It is a watchdog agency tasked with the mandate to guard against international disease transmission.

Centers for Medicare and Medicaid Services (CMS): A federal agency within the Department of Health and Human Services that administers Medicare, Medicaid, and the State Children's Health Insurance Program.

consumer-driven health plans (CDHP): Health benefits plans that engage covered individuals in choosing their own health-care providers, managing their own health expenses, and improving their own health with respect to factors that they can control.

computer physician order entry (CPOE): A computer-based system in the hospital setting for writing orders for medication and treatment. CPOE eliminates the need for transcription and improves medical documentation. CPOE software may be bundled with decision support software that helps physicians make more informed choices in patient care.

community health center: Federally funded medical facilities designed to provide ambulatory health services to underserved populations in both rural and urban areas.

digital dashboard: A control panel used in the emergency department of a hospital to track and monitor patients.

digital signature: A mathematical scheme for demonstrating the authenticity of a digital message or document. A valid digital signature gives a recipient reason to believe that the message was created by a known sender and that it was not altered in transit. Digital signatures are commonly used for software distribution, financial transactions, and in situations such as health care, where it is important to detect forgery or tampering.

e-health: The delivery of health-care services that incorporates the use of information technology and fosters a collaborative environment between a patient and a provider, which includes sharing of information and interactive communication.

electronic health record (EHR): An aggregate electronic record of health-related information on an individual that conforms to nationally recognized interoperability standards and that can be created, managed, and consulted by authorized clinicians and staff across more than one health-care organization. The EHR includes patient demographics, progress notes, problems, medications, medical history, immunizations, laboratory data, and radiology reports and images.

eICU: A location that is removed physically from the intensive care unit in a hospital where physicians can monitor several ICUs at the same time. The eICU can be located within a hospital complex or off site miles away and is manned around the clock by intensive care doctors and nurses.

e-Patients: Empowered health-care consumers who take an active role in their health care, collaborate with their providers, and use all available digital communication technology including the Internet, e-mail, smartphones, personal health records, and other applications and tools to manage and monitor their health and the health of family members.

electronic prescribing (e-prescribing): Entering a prescription in a data entry system and generating that prescription electronically.

e-visit: An asynchronous online discussion between a clinician and a patient via the Internet in a secure environment for the purpose of resolving issues and answering questions between office visits.

electronic mail (e-mail): The exchange of digital messages across the Internet.

ED/ER: Emergency department/emergency room in a hospital.

flexible savings accounts (FSA): An FSA allows an employee to set aside a portion of his or her earnings to pay for qualified expenses most commonly for medical expenses. It is similar to a health savings account (HSA) or a health reimbursement account (HRA). However, while HSAs and HRAs are almost exclusively used as components of a consumer-driven health-care plan, medical FSAs are commonly offered with more traditional health plans. Paper forms or an FSA debit card, also known as a flexcard, may be used to access the account funds.

Food and Drug Administration (FDA): The US Federal Agency responsible for protecting the public health by assuring the safety, efficacy, and security of human and veterinary drugs, biological products, medical devices, food supply, and cosmetics.

gatekeeper: A professional health-care provider who oversees and coordinates care for patients. That person could be a primary care physician, nurse practitioner, or physician assistant.

HapMap: Describes the common patterns of human DNA sequence variation. The HapMap database is a key resource for researchers to use to find genes affecting health, disease, and responses to drugs and environmental factors.

health information exchange (HIE): The electronic movement of health-related data and information, including e-mail, the Internet, digital databases, audio and video, among organizations according to specific standards, protocols, and other agreed criteria. (source: NAHIT)

health information technology (HIT): The deployment of digital communication tools, including e-mail, the Internet, digital databases, audio, and video, to facilitate information exchange among health-care providers and patients.

Health Insurance Portability Accountability Act (HIPAA): Legislation enacted in 1996 by the US Congress to protect health insurance coverage for workers and their families when they change or lose their job and to define national standards for electronic health-care transactions and address the privacy and security of health data.

health maintenance organization (HMO): An organization that provides health-care coverage in the United States through hospitals, doctors, and other providers with which the HMO has a contract. The HMO covers only care rendered by those doctors and other professionals who have agreed to treat patients in accordance with the HMO's guidelines and restrictions in exchange for a steady stream of customers.

health practice shortage area (HPSA): A region in the United States where there is a shortage of primary care physicians, dentists, and mental health practitioners as defined by CMS.

health-care payers: Insurers, including health plans, self-insured employer plans, and third party administrators, providing health-care benefits to enrolled members and reimbursing provider organizations.

health reimbursement accounts (HRA): Funds that a set aside by an employer on behalf of an employee for health-care needs.

health savings accounts (HSA): Funds set up to assist individuals with payment of out-of-pocket health expenses. Both employers and employees contribute to the HSA up to an annual amount limit set by statutory cap.

Hill-Burton Act of 1946: Provided funds to states for the construction of hospitals.

ICE (in case of emergency): An acronym that denotes an emergency contact who can be reached and who has access to an individual's electronic health record when that individual arrives in the emergency department unconscious and unable to communicate with the doctors.

Institute of Medicine (IOM): One of the United States' National Academies, IOM is a not for profit nongovernmental organization whose purpose is to provide advice on a variety of issues related to biomedical science, medicine and health. Each IOM report is reviewed by an expert panel that includes physicians, scientists, and others.

Medicare: A social insurance program administered by the United States government, providing health insurance coverage to people who are aged sixty-five and over.

medigap: Refers to private insurance plans sold to Medicare beneficiaries that provide coverage for medical expenses not or only partially covered by Medicare.

meaningful use: The meaningful use rules were established by the Center for Medicare and Medicaid Services and are used to define the criteria for payment to physicians under the American Recovery and Reinvestment Act of 2009. Meaningful use practice refers to health-care providers who use their electronic health records to engage patients and their families to take part in health-care decisions so that care coordination is improved and the privacy and security of health information remains intact. Meaningful use obliges health-care providers to reduce health-care disparities and improve population and public health.

National Health Information Network (NHIN): An initiative for the exchange of health-care information being developed under the auspices of the US Office of the National Coordinator for Health Information Technology (ONC).

nurse practitioners: Individuals who are licensed to practice medicine, to see patients, give exams, make diagnoses, make referrals, and treat acute illness, injuries, and infections, as well as prescribe medicine.

ONC: This is an acronym for the Office of the National Coordinator for Health Information Technology under the auspices of the Secretary of the Department of Health and Human Services. The national coordinator serves as the secretary's principal advisor on the development, application, and use of health information technology in an effort to improve the quality, safety, and efficiency of the nation's health through the development of an interoperable harmonized health information infrastructure.

patient-centered medical home (PCMH): An approach to providing comprehensive primary care that encourages collaboration between individual patients and their personal providers, and when appropriate, the patient's family. The PCMH becomes the main source of care for the patient.

patient portal: A secure website set up by a medical institution or a clinical practice where patients and doctors can maintain two-way password protected communication and where access to an electronic health record enables the patient/provider team to review medications, medical history, lab results, treatment programs, and other aspects of a patient's care.

Patient Protection and Affordable Care Act (PPACA): The Patient Protection and Affordable Care Act is a federal law that was signed by President Barack Obama on March 23, 2010. This act, along with the Health Care and Education Reconciliation Act of 2010 (signed into law on March 30, 2010) focuses on reform of the private health insurance market and includes provisions that provide improved coverage for those with preexisting conditions. It also addresses prescription drug coverage in Medicare and extends the life of the Medicare trust fund.

pay for performance (P4P): A payment approach used in health care that correlates payment to a physician with how well the physician adheres to practice standards and achieves certain outcomes based on a set of performance measures.

personal health record: An electronic cumulative record of health-related Information on an individual drawn from multiple sources that is created and managed by the individual. The data in the PHR and control of access to it are the responsibility of the individual.

Pew Internet and American Life Project: An initiative of the Pew Research Center, a nonprofit "fact tank" funded by the Pew charitable trusts founded by Joseph Pew. The Pew Internet and American Life Project provides information on the issues, attitudes, and trends with a particular focus on the impact of the internet on children, families, communities, the workplace, schools, health care, and civic/political life.

physician assistant (PA): A health-care professional licensed to practice medicine, with the supervision of a licensed physician, who works with patients in prevention, maintenance, and treatment, particularly individuals with chronic conditions. PAs conduct exams, order and interpret tests, counsel on preventive care, prescribe medicine, and sometimes assist in surgery.

point of service plan (POS): A managed-care health insurance system where patients are required to choose a primary care physician from an approved network to monitor their health care in exchange for a lower cost for their insurance.

preferred provider organization (PPO): A managed care organization of medical doctors, hospitals, and other health-care providers who have entered into an agreement with an insurer or a third-party administrator to provide health care at reduced rates to the insurer's or administrator's clients or patients.

primary care physician: A clinician who provides integrated health-care services and who addresses a large majority of personal health-care needs of patients in a sustained long-term relationship.

privacy rule: Legislation enacted by the US Congress in 2003 to establish the first federal privacy standards to protect patient health information.

Nancy B. Finn

protected health information: (PHI): Any information that concerns the health status, provision of health care, or payment for health care that can be linked to an individual.

provider: Any registered health professional who administers care to a patient. This can also refer to health-care delivery organizations.

registries: Organized systems for the collection, storage, retrieval, analysis, and dissemination of information about individual to support health needs. This also includes government agencies and professional associations that define, develop, and support registries.

regional health information organization (RHIO): A health information organization that brings together health-care stakeholders within a defined geographic area and governs health information exchange among them for the purpose of improving health and care in that community.

retail clinic: A medical facility, generally located at a retail pharmacy or other walk-in center (no appointment required), where patients can receive basic health-care services during regular hours as well as evenings and weekends. Fees for services are generally paid by the patient and are comparable to a standard co-payment.

radio frequency identification (RFID): Automatic identification based on radio waves, using devices called RFID tags or transponders that include an integrated circuit for storing and processing information and an antenna for receiving and transmitting the signal. RFID is used in health care to match patients with medication and to track materials and people within the health-care setting.

robots: Mechanical devices that include the software to make them capable of performing a variety of complex tasks such as measuring blood pressure, heart rate, and body temperature or inspecting incisions and performing surgical tasks. These robots are monitored and assisted by a physician.

specialist: A health-care provider who is trained in a specific area of medicine and offers care in that particular branch of medicine.

smart card: Similar to an ATM or credit card, it contains a patient's complete health history, including medications, insurance data, providers' names, and family history.

smartphone: A mobile phone that includes advanced connectivity and communication functionality, which is based on an operating software system that enables a great variety of applications. Among these applications are full Internet access, e-mail connectivity, cameras and video cameras, GPS systems, and audio features that enable the user to dictate notes into the device that can be transmitted to an electronic health record or stored and saved or other storage medium. Other applications include use as an MP3 player, an e-book reader, movie viewer, and more.

telemedicine: The use of communication equipment to link health-care practitioners and patients who are in different locations, allowing patients to receive care where and when it is needed. Telemedicine incorporates videoconferencing, the transmission of images, the use of patient portals, remote monitoring of vital signs, continuing medical education, and nursing call centers.

telerehabilitation/teletherapy: The clinical application of consultative preventative and therapeutics services via interactive telecommunication systems.

telemonitoring: Home health care using various digital devices and noninvasive wearable monitors that measure blood pressure, blood glucose, weight, and heart rate and send these measurements through a telephone system or through a computer to a remote site where medical providers can check the readings and take appropriate action.

Acknowledgments

Many individuals including physicians, nurses, nurse practitioners, hospital administrators, academics, technologists, commentators, and especially patients contributed thoughts, ideas and input for this book. These individuals helped because they believe in participatory medicine, patient empowerment, and healthcare delivery supported by digital communication technology that enables us to experience healthcare systems that are more efficient, effective and economical than the medical practices of the paper-based 20th century.

I owe a special thanks for their personal interest and mentoring of this project to: Dr. Joseph Kvedor Founder and Director of the Center for Connected Health at Partners Healthcare, Dr. Dan Teres, Medical Director at AstraZeneca, and Professor of Medicine at Tufts University Medical School, Dr. Danny Sands, assistant clinical professor of medicine at Harvard Medical School and senior medical informatics director for Cisco Systems Inc., Susannah Fox, Associate Director Digital Strategy Pew Internet and American Life Project, John Glaser, Chief Executive Officer of Siemens Health Services Business Unit. and former CIO of Partners Healthcare, Dr. Dena Pushkin, Director, Federal Office for the Advancement of Telehealth, U.S. Department of Health and Human Services, Michele Garvin, Esq. Ropes and Gray LLP, Dr. William F. Bria, Chief Medical Information Officer at Shiners Hospitals for Children.

Other individuals who contributed invaluable information include:

Susan A. Abookire, MD, MPH, Chair of Quality and Safety Medicine, Mount Auburn Hospital, Cambridge, MA.

Patricia Abbott, PhD, RN, Associate Professor and Co—Director WHO PAHO Collaborating Center for Nursing Knowledge Information Management and Sharing, Johns Hopkins University School of Medicine.

Thomas Abrams, Director, Division of Drug Marketing, Advertising, and Communications (DDMAC). Food and Drug Administration.

Holt Anderson, Executive Director, North Carolina Health Information and Communications Alliance.

Nina Antonetti, Telemedicine Manager, Marshfield Clinic Telehealth.

Dr. Peter Basch MD Senior Fellow. Center for American Progress, Director, Med Star Health, General Internist.

John Blair, MD, President & CEO, Taconic IPA.

William F. Bria, CMIO Shriners Hospitals for Children.

William Braithwaite, MD, PhD, FACMI, HISPI Vice Chairman, Health Information Policy Consultant.

Claire Broome MD,Former Director Integrated Health Information Systems, Centers for Disease Control and Prevention, Adjunct Professor Department of Global Health, Emery University School of Public Health.

Todd Brown, Associate Clinical Specialist and Vice Chair, Department of Pharmacy Practice, School of Pharmacy, Northeastern University.

Gary Christopherson, MD, Senior Advisor; Undersecretary for Health, Veterans Administration Senior Fellow, Institute of Medicine.

Homer L. Chin, MD, Medical Director, Clinical Information Systems, Kaiser Permanente.

David C. Classen, MD Vice President, First Consulting Group.

Jeffrey Cooper PhD, Director of biomedical engineering, Partners Healthcare, Boston MA.

Ted Cooper, MD. Associate Clinical Professor of Ophthalmology, Stanford University Medical School

Robert Cox, MD, Director Hays Medical Center, Hays Kansas.

Eliot Cutler, Director, Blood Lab at New England Medical Center, Boston.

Thomas Delbanco, MD Richard Florence Koplow-James Tullis Professor of General Medicine and Primary Care, Harvard Medical School, Founder, Division of General Medicine and, Primary Care Medicine Beth Israel Deaconess Medical Center, Boston, MA.

Suzanne Delbanco, Ph.D. founder and Executive Director of Catalyst for Payment Reform, formerly of The Leapfrog Group.

Henry DePhillips MD Chief Medical Officer, Medem.

George Demetri, MD, Director of Center for Sarcoma and Bone Oncology Dana Farber Cancer Institute, Associate Professor of Medicine Harvard Medical School.

Don E. Detmer, MD, President and CEO American Medical Informatics Association.

Joyce DuBow, Associate Director, AARP Public Policy.

David Ellis, MD, Associate Clinical Professor of Emergency Medicine, University of Buffalo

Ross D. Fletcher, MD, Chief of Staff VA Medical Center, Washington DC.

Mark Foster MD, Vice Chairman Taconic IPA Inc., Chairman THINC RHIO.

Charles Ganley, *M.D.*, Director. Division of Over-the-Counter Drug Products.FDA.

JanLori Goldman Columbia Health Privacy Project.

John Halamka, MD, MS, Chief Information Officer Caregroup Health System, Chief Information Officer, Harvard Medical School.

Claus Hamann Md. MS FRCP(C) Geriatric Primary Care Massachusetts General Hospital.

Matthew R. Handley, MD, Primary Care, Family Practice, Group Health Cooperative Seattle, WA.

Dan Hoch, MD, Department of Neurology, Massachusetts General Hospital.

Carol Holquist RPh, Director Division of Medication Errors and Technology Support, FDA, Washington, D.C.

David Jacobson, Professor of Anthropology, Brandeis University.

Joel Kahn MD, President, WorldCare Global Health Plan.

David W. Kaplan, MD,MPH, Chief Medical Information Officer, Children's Hospital, and Professor of Pediatrics, University of Colorado School of Medicine.

Charles M. Kilo, MD, MPH, Greenfield Health, Portland OR.

Bernard Koucher, MD, Founder, *Doctors without Borders.*

Howard M. Landa, MD, Kaiser Permanente Department of Pediatric Urology.

Thomas F. Landholt, MD, Family Practice, Springfield, MO.

David J. Lansky, PhD, President and CEO Pacific Business Group on Health, Former Senior Director Health Programs at the Markle Foundation.

Mark Leavitt MD, PhD Chairman of the Certification Commission for Healthcare. Information Technology (CCHIT).

Eric M. Liederman, MD MPH, Director of Medical Informatics, Kaiser Permanante UC Davis, Health Systems.

Steven R. Levisohn MD, Internal Medicine, Massachusetts General Hospital, Boston, MA.

Janet Marchibroda, Chief Healthcare Officer Global Healthcare and Life Sciences, IBM, Founder, eHealth Initiative.

Robert J. Mandel MD, MBA eHealth Program, Blue Cross Blue Shield, Massachusetts.

Bradford Middleton, MD, MPH, Chair Clinical Informatics, Research and Development, Clinical Informatics Research Department at Partners Healthcare.

David Nash MD, MBA Professor and Chairman of Health Policy, Thomas Jefferson University Medical College, Philadelphia, PA.

Larry Nathanson MD, Director Emergency Medicine Informatics, Beth Israel Deaconess Medical Center, Boston, MA.

Marc Overhage, MD, President and CEO of the Indiana Health Information Exchange.

David Rattner, MD, Chief of Division of Gastrointestinal and General Surgery, Massachusetts General Hospital.

Brian Rosenfeld, MD, Founder VISICU Inc.

David Rose, Chief Executive at Vitality and Founder of Ambient Devices.

Steve Ross, MD, Associate Professor University of Colorado Health Science Center, General Internal Medicine, University of Colorado Hospital.

Jay H. Sanders, M.D. President and CEO of the Global Telemedicine Group, Professor of Medicine at Johns Hopkins University School of Medicine.

Joseph Scherger, MD, MPH, Professor of Clinical Family and Preventive Medicine at the University of California, San Diego School of Medicine.

Steve L. Schneider MD Associate Director, Healthwise, Co-founder Idaho Wellness Center.

Hasan Sharif MD, Founder, COO, CMO, WorldCare.

Linda E. Silvers, Health Fraud Team, U.S. Food and Drug Administration.

Warner Slack, MD, Department Neurology, Beth Israel Deaconess Medical Center, Boston, MA.

Joseph Siemienszuk, MD, CMO Providence Health System.

Paul Tang, MD, MS, Vice President and Chief Medical Information Officer Palo Alto Medical Foundation (PAMF). Stanford CA.

Lisa Vetter Telemedicine Specialist St. Alexius Medical Center North Dakota.

Jonathan S. Wald, MD, MPH Former Associate Director of the Clinical Informatics Research and Development (CIRD) Group Partners Healthcare, Director PC Technology at RTI International.

Kenneth Weiss, PHD. Psychologist and Clinical Instructor, Harvard Medical School.

Andrew Wiesenthal, MD, Associate Executive Director for Clinical Information Support The Permanente Federation.

David Williams Principal, MedPharma Partners LLC.

Eric Zimmerman, Senior Vice President, Relay Health.

Special thanks to my graphic artist, Tania Helhoski of Bird Design and to Ed Shems, a talented illustrator who did the cartoons that appear in the book. My grateful appreciation to Maureen Doherty, Mim and Mark Goldberg, Robin Jaeger and Dr. Rachel Wulf Silver who spent many hours reviewing the book, and finally everlasting appreciation to my husband Peter Finn whose patience, insights and sense of humor made it possible for me to enjoy and complete this project.

Index

D
Daily Strength, 137
diabetes, 129–130
digital dashboards, 56–57, 190
digital health records.
      See electronic health
      records (EHR); personal
      health records (PHR)
digital signature, 190
DNA sequencing, 183
doctors
   choosing of, 72
   communication with, 1–9, 64
   primary care providers, 94, 175, 195
Dossia, 18
drugs, 133–134
      See also pharmacies, online

E
Early Retiree Reinsurance Program
      (ERRP), 175–176
e-health, 190
eICU, 88, 91, 182, 191
electronic health records (EHR),
      2, 5, 12–16, 25, 145, 152,
      189, 190
electronic prescribing, 2, 69–70, 191
e-mail
   benefits of, 31–32
   and chronic conditions, 30, 41
   and continuous care, 28–31
   defined, 191
   etiquette for, 32–33, 40
   privacy of, 32–33, 41
emergency contacts, 39, 41, 55, 193
emergency rooms (ER), 55–57, 191
e-Patients, xi–xiv, 7–8, 9, 191
e-prescribing, 2, 69–70, 191

etiquette, 32–33, 40
e-visits, 33, 35, 102–107, 112, 191

F
Facebook, 136
family history, 134
familydoctor.org, 125
fee-for-service insurance, 164
Ferguson, Tom, xii
Fibrohugs, 117–118
fibromyalgia, 117–118
flexible spending accounts (FSA),
      170, 191

G
gatekeeper, 63, 94, 183, 191
glossary, 189–197
Google Health, 123–124, 148
Group Loop, 139

H
HapMap, 182, 192
health care
   costs of, 89, 158–161, 184–185
   future of, 178–180, 183–186
   major trends in, 188
   plan choices, 161–170
   poor performance of, 160–161
health information exchange
      (HIE), 24–25, 156, 192
health information technology
      (HIT), 186, 192
health insurance, 18, 161–172
Health Internet Ethics, 120
health maintenance organization
      (HMO), 165–166, 192

of the future, 182
for the greater good, 89–90
and health care costs, 89
legal issues, 82–83
mental health services, 80
physical therapy, 79
second opinion consults, 82
speech therapy, 77
telehospice, 81
teletherapy, 77, 197
telemonitoring, 83, 197
telerehabilitation, 90, 197
telestroke centers, 81
teletherapy, 77, 197
travelers' health, 132–133
Twitter, 136–137

U
US Food and Drug Administration
(FDA), 133–134
US Justice Department, 151–152
USB memory sticks, 19

V
Veterans Administration (VA),
21–23, 24–25, 71, 150

W
Wasson, Susan Rutten, 107–108
web portal sites. *See* patient portals
WebMD, 18, 126, 148
websites
about cardiac and lung diseases, 130
about consumer information
services, 122–123
about diabetes, 129–130

about fibromyalgia, 117–118
about general health and
wellness, 125–126, 176
about HIV, 131
about patient safety, 71
about prescription drugs, 71,
133–134
about traveling, 132–133
about weight loss, 131–132
for cancer patients, 128–129, 139
credibility of, 119–121
for finding doctors and
hospitals, 126–127
gateway sites, 123–125
of medical institutions, 127–128
of professional organizations, 128
recommended, 122–123, 141
for social networking, 135–140
See also Internet
weight loss, 131–132
Whalen v. Roe, 154–155

Y
Yahoo Health, 124
yourdiseaserisk.com, 125